What Every Parent Should Know
About Childhood Immunization

What Every Parent Should Know About Childhood Immunization

JAMIE MURPHY

EARTH HEALING PRODUCTS
BOSTON

Requests for permissions should be mailed to:
Permissions, Earth Healing Products, P.O. Box 11, Dennis, Massachusetts 02638

First Printing 1993
Second Printing 1994
Third Printing 1994
Fourth Printing 1995
Fifth Printing 1997
Sixth Printing 1998

Library of Congress Catalog Card Number 91-092500
ISBN 0-9630373-0-7

Editor: Carol White
Cover design: Meryl Brenner
Typesetting: Tom Hathcoat
Cover photo: Copyright © Elizabeth Crews/Stock Boston
Text printed on recycled paper
Printed in the United States of America

Permissions granted to the author appear on page 180.

Contents

CHAPTER 1

What Every Parent Should Know

C hildhood immunization is one of the least understood subjects in the field of medicine, yet it is one of crucial importance. It is least understood by parents and other laypeople because we have rarely questioned its validity.

For almost two hundred years the majority of people have accepted that vaccines are necessary for the health and safety of their children. But where did such a strong belief originate? I believe that much of the acceptance for immunization has been conditioned by state laws, which dictate that children receive vaccines for polio, diphtheria, pertussis, tetanus, measles, mumps, rubella, and, in some states, hemophilus influenzae, before they are allowed to attend school. I also believe that we have accepted immunizations primarily on the recommendations of physicians, who almost uniformly advocate them, yet who minimize the extent of adverse reactions, in some cases refusing to believe that a direct connection exists between immunization and a serious reaction to it.

Most people learn about immunization when they bring their two-month old infant to a health clinic or family pediatrician for vaccination shots. Unfortunately, most parents leave the doctor's office with a screaming baby cradled in their arms and only a vague understanding of what just happened. Few physicians explain to parents what immunizations are, how they work, what protections they give, and what short- or long-term side effects can occur. When concerned parents ask their doctors about the safety of vaccines, most are given a routine answer, "The benefits outweigh the risks."

Almost all the literature pertaining to vaccination that appears in medical journals, encyclopedias, and high school and college textbooks heralds it as one of the great medical discoveries of the nineteenth century. Since 1988 I have researched scores of vaccination documents in public and medical school libraries and have spoken with parents of vaccine-damaged children. After reviewing the historical, medical, legal, and chemical aspects of immunization, I have come to the conclusion that vaccines are dangerous to one's health, and that the risks clearly outweigh the benefits.

What Every Parent Should Know about Childhood Immunization explores the magnificent role our immune system plays in protecting us from infection and disease. It also outlines the differences between natural and artificial immunity and investigates the impact vaccines have on our infants' immune systems and health. I hope that it does this in language you will understand in order that we might come closer to answering a crucial question: Are vaccines really necessary? In addition, the book examines the protective qualities of breast milk in which antibodies to all the inoculable childhood diseases have been found. More importantly, perhaps, you will learn the little-known ways to legally avoid immunizations for your children.

What Every Parent Should Know about Childhood Immunization is a comprehensive look at the rarely discussed secretive and mysterious aspects of immunization—how vaccines are created in the laboratory, toxic chemicals used in the vaccines, and the role animal experimentation plays in their production. Lastly, the book uncovers the adverse side effects and long-term conditions vaccines may have caused and how frequently the DPT vaccine produces local, systemic, and neurological reactions in infants and children.

The decision to vaccinate or not to vaccinate your child is one of the most important health decisions you will make in your lifetime. In the past, for many, that decision has been made with only a fraction of the considerations necessary to arrive at an informed choice. It is my sincere hope that the information contained in this book will help you make that choice and guide you to what is best for you and your child.

CHAPTER 2

The Power
of Human Immunity

*B*efore we can determine whether immunization is necessary
for infants and children, we need to define what vaccines
are and observe the role they play in human immunity. Vaccines
are treated preparations containing bacteria or viruses that are
used to artificially induce immunity against a specific disease. A
vaccine is designed to mimic the process of naturally occurring
infection by artificial means. Theoretically, a vaccine produces
in recipients a mild episode of infection, whose side effects,
though common, are supposed to be slight and from which
infants and children are supposed to recover easily. The aim of
vaccination is to prevent full-blown clinical disease or the type
of disease children would theoretically contract if they were not
vaccinated—provided of course that their living standard,
hygiene, acquired immunity, maternal care, and reservoirs of
natural immunity all failed them.

The agent in the vaccine that stimulates immunity is called
the antigen. Bacteria, viruses, pollen, fungi, protozoans, and
poisons from insects and snakes are all antigens. An antigen is
any substance that, when introduced into the body, stimulates
the production of antibodies. Antibodies are various proteins
that circulate in the blood and are produced in response to an
antigen. Antibodies are beneficial to us and are a key element
in our immune defense. The antibody's mission in life is to
neutralize antigens, thereby keeping the blood clear of foreign
invaders.

Essentially, vaccination promises protection against a select
number of diseases that, for some mysterious reason, our own
immune system and natural health resources cannot deal with
effectively on their own. Vaccines are portrayed as being

indispensible and somehow better at disease protection than what our innate biological defenses and nutritional resources have accomplished for thousands of years. Could this be possible?

The decision to vaccinate a child is often made without considering that we have the power and strength of our own natural immunity to protect us from illness. It is upon the foundation of natural immunity that people have overcome infection and disease, to a lesser or greater degree, since time immemorial. While so much has already been written in books and medical texts in praise of natural immunity (i.e., our ability to withstand and overcome infections, diseases, and self-heal), all of that becomes overshadowed or forgotten every time a physician injects a vaccine into a child. Therefore, in order to weigh the strengths and weaknesses of artificial immunity or the type induced by vaccination, we must first observe the magnificent role our immune system plays in defending against potentially harmful disease states. The following discussion outlines some of the most important ways we resist infection and disease.

NATURAL IMMUNITY

Nature gives all creatures of the earth distinct ways to function and survive in the world. Birds, insects, and mammals each have their own unique way of finding food, building a home, and providing for their young. Similarly, nature provides an important biological function that animals and humans share, the ability to resist infection and disease. This is called natural immunity.

In humans, natural immunity might be defined as the sum total of our inherent biological immune defenses that are not artificially induced. Natural resistance to infection is a relative state of immunity that does not depend on being previously exposed to an antibody-producing substance (antigen) in order to gain protection. An example of this capability is found in lysozyme, an enzyme present in saliva and tears, which dissolves microbes. A further example of natural resistance is our skin, which provides a physical barrier against microbes and has the capacity for rapid healing of cuts and scrapes.

The ability to resist disease and overcome infection is one of the major attributes of human immunity. However, because people express their resistance to illness differently (i.e, as mild, moderate, or severe reactions, and many times with no symptoms at all), simple definitions of "healthy" and "sick" can become obscured.

Studies on the prevalence of poliomyelitis provide a good example of how individuals show different levels of resistance to this disease. It is well known that many children harbor the polio virus in their intestine yet never get paralytic polio. In fact, most cases of polio exist as subclinical infections, that is, without any noticeable symptoms.[1] In other cases, symptoms such as severe headaches, malaise, and neck pain occur. Most individuals recover from this form of polio after a short period of time, without any complications. A third reaction to the polio virus, and the one least frequent, is paralytic polio. This occurs when the virus passes beyond the protective barriers of the intestinal mucosa and lymph nodes and invades the central nervous system, attacking motor neurons in the brain stem and spinal cord. Epidemiologists estimate that the polio virus enters the central nervous system in only 1 of every 1,000 cases.[2] Even if this happens, paralytic polio may or may not ensue. It appears that paralysis is permanent only when there is a complete destruction of the nerve cells.[3]

Polio is a common infection in some tropical areas of the world, where the native people encounter it as a frequent non-threatening illness.[4] When outsiders visit these countries, some become infected with full-blown clinical symptoms. Where is their natural resistance to polio? It appears that early exposure to it or repeated subclinical infections build resistance to polio in the native people. This process of gaining immunity is called acquired resistance. When visitors encounter the polio virus, usually as adults and perhaps for the first time, some are vulnerable to it because they have not developed a stronger response to the virus, after repeated "small doses" of it.[5]

Acquired resistance, however, is not the only factor that determines the outcome of an encounter with an infectious agent. There are many underlying mechanisms of disease resistance, some well known, and others in need of further study. These include factors such as: heredity, race, environmental factors, the effect of climate, and nutrition. Resistance may also be unique to a particular species. Cattle and sheep can contract foot and mouth disease while humans are largely immune. Similarly, many animals successfully avoid diphtheria, yet children are susceptible.[6]

Whether resistance is innate or acquired, the protection that nature gives us is not absolute and invariably conforms to the way we nourish our bodies with food and our being with love and self-acceptance. In particular, among other factors, the relative nutritional and emotional health of an individual is a significant factor that influences the level of our resistance to infection and disease.

Types of Immunity

Human immunity can be innate or it can be acquired, actively or passively, naturally or artificially. Innate immunity refers to the biological protections that we are born with or inherit.

Active immunity is acquired naturally when microorganisms begin to colonize the intestinal and respiratory tract of the infant. Active immunity is acquired artificially through immunization, with dead or living organisms (antigens) from the vaccine.

Passive immunity is acquired naturally when maternal antibodies pass from mother to fetus (through the blood circulation) during pregnancy and from the mother's breast milk after birth. Passive immunity is acquired artificially when immune serum (containing antibodies from animals or humans) is administered to an individual.

The human immune system is a complex network of blood proteins, chemicals, tissues, hormones, and organs, which collectively protect us from foreign invaders and disease. Because the immune system is so vast, it is difficult to say where one aspect of it begins and another ends. In spite of the complexity of the immune system, science has been able to untangle many of its functions and present them in stages, as a first, second, and third line of defense. It is these lines of defense which provide natural body protections from antigens.

Immunologists have been able to further classify our immune response to harmful germs (within the overlapping parameters of a first, second, and third line of defense), as being either specific or non-specific. Although difficult to categorize, non-specific immune response or immunity refers to all the ways the body mounts its offense and defense against foreign invaders, as distinguished from the singular antibody-antigen reaction known as specific immunity. The skin, the digestive and respiratory mucous membranes and their secretions, the act of coughing, sneezing reflexes, sweating, fever, natural antibodies, the inflammatory response, proteins called complement and interferon, fatty acids, R-E cells, and the devouring of antigens by phagocytes (in a process known as phagocytosis) are all examples of non-specific immune responses.

In the pages that follow many examples of non-specific immune responses are given. Some are first line defenses, while others probably fit more readily as second line. Because the immune system operates as an integrated organism with many of its functions overlapping, interrelating, and involving all three levels of defense, categories become obsured and ultimately are not that important. Nevertheless, with a little bit of imagination, we can visualize how potentially dangerous microbes are dealt with and trace their pathway, more or less, from their port of entry on through to the bloodstream.

FIRST LINE OF DEFENSE: THE SKIN AND BODY FLORA

The skin and the secretions of the mucous membranes form the first line of defense against pathogens. The skin acts as a physical barrier and produces chemicals that prevent the entry of microbes into the body. The outer layer of skin contains a proteinous material called keratin, which provides a tough resilient cover.[7] Chemical secretions, such as fatty acids and lactic acids produced from oily sebaceous glands and from sweating, further inhibit the growth of bacteria on the skin.[8]

Although bacteria are usually portrayed as villains, capable of destroying tissue and polluting the body, most bacteria are harmless when they are kept in place by the body's natural barriers. The vast majority of bacteria that live on or in our body are beneficial to us and cooperate in maintaining our health. The microorganisms that populate parts of our skin, ears, mouth, throat, urinary system, and colon are known collectively as the body flora.[9] The flora consists of bacteria and other microorganisms known as commensals. The term commensal means "sharing the same table, eating the same food source." Commensals feed on surface cells and are otherwise not harmful. They may perform beneficial functions such as digesting waste products in the intestinal tract and assisting in the production of certain vitamins such as Vitamin K (blood-clotting vitamin) and Vitamin B12 (anti-anemic vitamin).[10]

Many varieties of bacteria live inside us without causing disease. Although potentially dangerous microbes inhabit the intestinal and respiratory tract of healthy people, infection does not occur.[11] Typhoid germs spread on the skin will die more quickly than those spread equally on a glass plate. The bacteria streptococcus viridians lives rather unobtrusively in our mouth, yet the toxin it excretes is capable of causing endocarditis, a bacterial infection affecting the heart.[12] Another bacteria called hemophilus influenza type B resides in our throat without causing any obvious harm, yet this organism has been implicated as the cause of a virulent type of meningitis that affects children.[13]

While the exact mechanism by which the flora prevents infection is not known, it is thought that these commensals may produce waste products which become food for some microorganisms, while at the same time inhibiting the growth of others.[14] If beneficial flora are present, they keep out more harmful or pathogenic microbes. The flora contributes greatly to our health by providing checks and balances among organisms.

The beneficial role of the flora becomes most evident when we observe the destructive changes antibiotics deliver to the flora and its ecosystem.

Antibiotics are drugs often derived from bacteria and fungi which are used to combat bacterial growth or infection. While they are effective against harmful bacteria, they are also destructive to the beneficial commensals. When penicillin is administered to treat mouth or throat infections caused by streptococci or pneumococci germs, it will effectively destroy disease-causing organisms. However, antibiotics are indiscriminate and destroy harmless or beneficial bacteria as well.

Antibiotics that fight bacteria are ineffective against the yeast organism candida albicans, a commensal which lives in our throat and other areas of the body. Because friendly organisms that ordinarily hold the growth of candida albicans in check are killed by penicillin, the candida yeast grows out of control.[15] Other drugs such as steroids, contraceptives, immunosuppressives (used after organ transplants), and cytotoxics (anti-cancer drugs) can disturb the flora and allow for an overgrowth of candida, leading to infections such as oral candidiasis (thrush), urinary tract infections, or vulvovaginitis, a condition suffered by women and characterized by a yellow-whitish discharge with inflammation of the vaginal wall.[16,17] The use of antibiotics over an extended period can obliterate friendly bacterial colonies in the bowel, resulting in diarrhea or bleeding.[18] In fact, repeated rounds of antibiotics, given to fight bacterial infection, can ultimately weaken the body's ability to withstand other infections as well. Clearly, the health and maintenance of the body flora is a vital non-specific defense and needs to be protected or replaced when antibiotics, steroids, or birth control pills disrupt their presence.

More Body Protections

While the skin and the body flora provide protection from unwanted pathogens, other non-specific defenses provide additional first and second line protection. Lysozyme, an enzyme found in tears, saliva, and other body fluids is destructive to certain kinds of bacteria. Small hairs called cilia, found on the surface of mucosal cells in the respiratory tract, sweep dust and bacterial particles upward, away from the lungs. When the debris reaches the throat, it is either swallowed or expelled by coughing. Coughing and sneezing remove a great deal of trapped dust, bacteria, and virus particles from the respiratory tract. The stomach lining produces hydrochloric acid, which is powerful enough to kill many microbes. Other secretions in the respiratory tract contain antibodies called secretory immunoglobulin which help white blood cells ingest pathogenic organisms.[19]

Natural Antibodies

Antibodies are proteins found in the blood that protect us from foreign invaders. They are usually formed in direct response to a specific antigen, either from a naturally occurring infection or from a self-induced attack via immunization.

Natural antibodies are serum proteins produced "in the absence of an environmental stimulation."[20] There seems to be some speculation about how natural antibodies could escape exposure to an antigen. One explanation asserts that natural antibodies might receive their stimulation from a "harmless" bacterium inside the body, after which the natural antibody becomes destructive to a second type of virulent bacteria.[21] Cells that secrete natural antibodies have been found in the spleen and are known to be produced throughout a lifetime.[22] In any event, their presence is another beneficial element of our natural immunity.

The Inflammatory Response

Another feature of non-specific immunity is the inflammatory response. When tissue is injured, either by irritation or infection, inflammation occurs, resulting in tenderness, redness, swelling, and pain. During an inflammation response, trauma to tissue cells sets off a remarkable series of events which protect us from further injury. First, connective tissue blocks the lymph channel to check the possible spread of invading microbes.[23] Next, the injured cells' capillaries become larger, enabling a more rapid flow of white blood cells called neutrophils from the blood stream through the capillary walls to the site of the injury.[24] An acute inflammation response calls forth other warriors such as: C-reactive protein, natural antibodies, IgM, interferon, properdin, and complement.[25] If microbes are able to penetrate the skin, the mucous membranes, the chemistries of the stomach, or the secretions of the intestine, they will encounter the body's second line of resistance, the lymphatic-circulatory system.

SECOND LINE OF DEFENSE: THE LYMPHATIC SYSTEM

The lymphatic system forms the second line of defense against pathogens. Lymph is a clear, colorless fluid, which acts as a filter for blood by removing wastes and dangerous elements. Cells are like islands surrounded by an ocean of lymph fluid. The lymphatic system filters and purges unwanted elements from the fluids that bathe the cells. The system consists of lymph nodes, lymphatic vessels, the spleen, and the thymus gland. Lymph flow is a passive process—it is dependent upon muscle contraction and is an important benefit of physical activity. The contraction of various muscles moves the lymph fluid through the lymph nodes, spleen, and thymus gland, filtering out debris and pathogens. The connective tissue within the glands and vessels of the lymphatic system contains the bacteria-devouring cells, the lymphocytes and macrophages. Eventually the lymph vessels collect into a larger vessel called the thoracic duct which reenters the general circulation near the heart. The liver and kidneys remove the wastes collected by the lymphatic vessels and purge them from the body.

The lymphatic system also contains a widely dispersed group of cells and tissues known as the reticulo-endothelial cells or R-E cells. R-E cells form the lining of the heart, spleen, liver, blood vessels, thymus gland, and lymph nodes. It is within the connective mesh of the lymph nodes that R-E cells trap and ingest microbes.[26] R-E cells in the liver and spleen also function as a filter for the blood that moves through its network of channels. R-E cells provide a vital, non-specific line of defense by keeping the blood and lymph free of pathogens.

The lymphatic system performs an integral role in defending the body from systemic infections. At the peak of microbial invasion, lymphocytes are mobilized to these sites to conduct a vital defense against pathogens.

Complement

Complement, found in blood, consists of liquid chemical or non-specific protein complexes that have a bactericidal action. Complement or the complement system is involved in complex immune processes that fix antibody to antigen on cell surfaces. Thus the presence of complement is indispensable for the destruction of bacteria by antibody.[27] Among other important functions, complement is involved in orchestrating the movement of certain white blood cells called neutrophils to the site of bodily injury or infection.

Interferon

Interferons, another important element of non-specific immunity, are proteins that are produced by cells already infected with viruses.[28] Viruses are able to replicate within a cell by controlling the cell's computer brain (DNA or RNA) and telling it to make more copies of the virus. Interferon disrupts this process by not allowing the viruses to multiply, thus blocking the movement of virus from infected cells to new cell hosts. The production of interferon also stimulates natural killer cells, which scientists believe have the ability to inhibit the growth of tumor cells.[29]

Scavenger Cells: Macrophages and Leukocytes

In 1884, Ilya Mechnikov, a Russian bacteriologist, discovered certain white blood cells which he called "microphages" and "macrophages." The names were derived from the Greek, meaning "little eaters" and "big eaters."[30] Mechnikov recognized that these cells had the ability to ingest and "dismantle" microbes found in the blood. While the name macrophages has not changed, microphages are now known as white blood cells or leukocytes.

Leukocytes are produced in the bone marrow and circulate freely in the bloodstream. Neutrophils are the most abundant type of leukocyte and are the first white blood cells to arrive at the site of an injury. In ways that are not entirely understood, bacteria and other pathogens adhere to neutrophil membranes before they are devoured. It is thought that blood proteins called opsonins coat bacteria with antibody, enabling the bacteria to stick more readily to the neutrophil cell body.[31] Neutrophils, sensing the coated bacterium (antigen), surround the germ by wrapping their membrane around it.[32] Lastly, neutrophils destroy the antigen with a powerful bactericidal enzyme. The disintegration and ingestion of the microbe is called phagocytosis.

The second type of scavenger cell is the macrophage. Macrophages are produced in the bone marrow and come in two varieties: monocytes and fixed tissue macrophages. Monocytes circulate freely in the blood and destroy pathogens directly.[33] Fixed macrophages are plentiful in the connective tissue of the spleen, lymph nodes, and the thymus gland. Among other important functions, fixed macrophages prepare antigens for their final elimination by the action of plasma cells.[34]

The Activation of Lymphocytes

After macrophages ingest bacteria or other unwanted cells, the processed antigens appear on the surface of their membranes.[35] White blood cells called T-cell lymphocytes sense the antigen determinants on the cell membranes and, in response, send out "chemical messages" known as lymphokines.[36] Lymphokines alert other cells called B-cell lymphocytes to produce antibody in response to the processed antigen. Antibody coats the antigen which is later ingested by scavenger cells called phagocytes. The activation of the lymphoctes brings into play the processes of specific immunity and the body's third line of defense.

THIRD LINE OF DEFENSE:
ANTIBODIES AND SPECIFIC IMMUNITY

Specific immunity refers to the protection given to us by immunoglobulins. Immunoglobulins are often referred to as antibodies and designated as Ig's. Antibodies are produced in response to a specific antigen. The memory of the interaction between antigen and antibody is the distinguishing feature of specific immunity. If or when the antigen in question invades the body again, the memory of the first encounter produces antibodies more rapidly the second time.

The B-cells are the first lymphocytes involved in specific immunity. They are produced in the bone marrow like red blood cells, yet their greatest concentration is in the tissue of the thymus gland, spleen, lymph nodes, tonsils, and the lining of the intestines.[37] B-cells are constrained in the mesh of connective tissue that directs lymphocytes toward foreign antigens trapped by macrophages. When B-cells are stimulated by an antigen, they are transformed into plasma cells. Plasma cells manufacture only one kind of antibody effective against only one antigen. Antibodies that are secreted by plasma cells circulate throughout the body fluids, blood, and lymph. The word "humor" is an old medical term used to describe the body fluids. Consequently, the immunity given to us by B-cells is called humoral immunity.

The Immunoglobulins

The antibodies secreted by the plasma cells are known collectively as the immunoglobulins (Ig's). There are five classes of immunoglobulins, each with an important job to accomplish.

IgM is the first antibody reproduced in response to a pathogen. It is a large molecule, usually found in the blood, which "stimulates" phagocytosis and "activates" complement.[38]

IgG is the most plentiful antibody in the bloodstream. It is transferred from mother to fetus during pregnancy, passing from maternal to fetal bloodstreams, bestowing passive immunity on the fetus and newborn. IgG activates macrophages and can trigger complement fixation. IgG kills antigens directly and is one of the antibodies that is churned out during a viral or bacterial attack.

IgA is found in the saliva, tears, sweat, tonsils, colostrum, and breast milk.[39] It is also produced by the mucosal cells in the respiratory, intestinal, and urinary tracts. IgA is primarily involved in local immunity to subdue or defeat microbes at the first line of defense.

IgE is the antibody involved with allergic reactions, such as hay fever or food allergies.

IgD is located in the blood, but only in small concentrations. It is also found on the surfaces of circulating B-lymphocytes, yet its role in immunity is not well defined.[40]

T-Cell Lymphocytes

The second type of lymphocyte involved in specific immune responses is the T-cell. T-cells originate in the bone marrow but mature in the thymus gland. After they are developed, T-cells circulate in the blood and lymph, yet unlike the plasma cells do not produce antibodies. The protection that T-cells provide is called cell-mediated immunity.

An important characteristic of T-cell lymphocytes is their capacity to "remember" an encounter with a germ or foreign element in the body. When T-cells encounter an antigen, they are able to distinguish it from millions of other foreign molecules. If that antigen should reappear, the memory of the former encounter produces T-cells faster and in greater numbers, before the immune system is overwhelmed by a bacterial or viral attack.

Some T-cells devour antigens directly, while others provide equally important functions. During a bacterial or viral invasion, the T-helper cells produce chemical "hormones," which alert other fighter cells that the conflict with antigens is beginning.[41] T-suppressor cells produce hormones which signal an end to the confrontation.[42]

Human beings have a natural resistance to disease. It is a miracle of life that is given to us. Our immune system is a wonderfully complex and powerful ally that protects us from potentially harmful bacteria and viruses by maintaining balance and order in our bodies. The integrated defenses of our immune system, our natural resistance to disease, and the strength we give ourselves in the form of nutritional sustenance are the primary reasons that we are able to withstand infection and heal ourselves.

We have seen that the body resists infection in many ways. Ivan Roitt, the author of *Essential Immunology* and a leading immunologist, reinforces a key point about the power and strength of human immunity: "The first contact with an infectious organism clearly imprints some memory, so that the body is effectively prepared to repel any later invasion by that organism."[43]

This concept is fundamental to human immunity. It is significant because it leads one to ask crucial questions: Why should we artificially provoke an immune reaction through vaccination when microorganisms in the environment do this anyway? Why should we even attempt to duplicate an essential biological process which nature has so wisely provided us? In short, why do we need immunization?

CHAPTER 3

Immunization Versus Natural Immunity

*B*oth vaccination and natural infection stimulate the production of antibody. During a natural infection pathogenic organisms may or may not reach the bloodstream. The entire spectrum of non-specific immune defenses, whose job is to protect host cells from pathogens and to destroy and eliminate antigens, provides a formidable defense in limiting the quantity of antigens that may eventually reach the bloodstream. Undoubtedly, our level of non-specific immune response influences the severity of the infection as well.

Because vaccines have a somewhat different impact on the immune system than natural infections, it is useful to make comparisons between the two events. Richard Moskowitz, M.D., author of *The Case Against Immunizations*, offers some valuable insights on the differences between measles and the measles vaccine.

MEASLES V. MEASLES VACCINE

Measles is an acute infectious disease of the respiratory tract that generally affects children. It is contagious through contact with infected viral materials in the air. The measles virus undergoes an incubation period of ten to fourteen days before symptoms are noticed. During the incubation period, the virus begins a journey that starts in the tonsils, moves to the lymph nodes and other lymphoid tissues, and finally passes into the spleen, blood, and other immune organs.[1] When symptoms of measles become noticeable, circulating antibodies are already present in the blood. One might view a person's reaction to the measles virus, such as swollen lymph glands and high antibody levels, as abnormal. Moskowitz, however, sees this situation as the natural response of the immune system to simply remove or filter the virus from the blood.[2] Other responses to the measles invasion are noteworthy. For one, much of the natural measles virus may be eliminated through coughing and sneezing, permitting the virus to be expelled from the same areas through which it tried to pass, the mouth, nose, and throat.[3] Furthermore, because measles is an acute disease, it will initiate a major response from the immune system, including many non-specific factors such as inflammatory response and the activation of macrophages, neutrophils, and complement.[4] In addition, the secretion of local antibody in the respiratory tract, called secretory Ig A, will help defeat the measles virus at its port of entry. Thus, aside from the unpleasant nature of having measles, undergoing the illness usually confers lifelong immunity to its recipients.

The benefits of experiencing measles must be seen in context; it is a large step toward developing the overall capacity of the child's immune system and for strengthening the ability to overcome other infections as well.

In contrast, the measles vaccine is injected into muscle tissue, which bypasses the normal port of entry for the virus, the mouth and nose, thus avoiding any possibility of eliminating virus or reducing the dose through coughing and sneezing. Second, because the virus has been attenuated, the vaccine product will neither provoke a major inflammatory response nor activate the necessary non-specific immune defenses.[5] Most importantly, by giving a child the measles vaccine, we have introduced the virus into the blood and "immune organs" for which it has an affinity, as Moskowitz says "with no obvious way to get rid of it."[6]

The production of circulating antibodies is the desired result of vaccination, for this is a strong indication that infection with vaccine virus has taken place. In one important study, which measured the level of circulating antibody in children, 10½ years after they received the combined measles, mumps, and rubella vaccine, all individuals had detectable antibodies in their blood to the three antigens.[7] The persistence of antibody in the blood of vaccinees gives assurance to the vaccinators that this induced vaccine immunity, which is never 100 percent effective to begin with, is still working. However, this kind of reasoning is unsubstantiated, as is evidenced by the number of booster shots that are needed to keep vaccine immunity current. In the case of measles vaccine, the argument can be made that artificial immunity is fleeting regardless of the presence of circulating antibody to the measles antigen. This is evident from epidemics of measles that have occurred in recent years (1983-1990) in which a substantial number of cases of measles have repeatedly occurred in children and young adults who had been fully vaccinated against measles, and whose serum revealed that they were immune to measles.[8]

The price we pay for artificial immunity of this sort is far greater than we can imagine, yet the issue is apparently of only academic interest to the medical profession. The production of antibodies via immunizations comes at a great cost, for in order to produce antibodies, we must have antigens continuously stimulating their production. Antigens—whether they come from measles virus in the environment or from a measles vaccine—are precisely what the entire immune system is geared to destroy and eliminate. Consequently, the reality of having vaccine antigens in our blood and tissues, for extended periods of time, raises some serious questions about vaccine use.

What is the safe quantity of vaccine antigens that will not cause local, systemic, and sometimes severe neurological damage in infants and children? What happens to vaccine antigens in the body years later? Where do they go and of what are they capable? What is the safe amount of vaccine antigen that will stimulate immunity but not cause disease? The answer to this last question is largely unknown, because there is no precise way to calculate that amount. Again, it would seem logical to make comparisons with natural infection, since immunizations are supposed to mimic the naturally occurring process. However, medical scientists do not know the infecting dose of a naturally occurring infection.[9] It is an unknown quantity, and an impractical experiment to perform, perhaps as futile as trying to measure the amount of sunlight it takes to make a plant grow.

Consequently, scientists test vaccines on animals, extrapolate the data, and apply the results to human beings.

While it is evident that scientists do not have an accurate model for determining the safe amount of antigen to use in a vaccine, we do know, by comparison, something extremely valuable about the infecting dose of a naturally occurring infection. Harold Buttram, M.D. and John Chriss Hoffman in their work *Vaccinations and Immune Malfunction*, point out that inapparent infections outnumber observable sickness by 100 to 1.[10] Inapparent infections, which are also known as subclinical infections, are insufficient to produce the normal, recognizable disease. Living proof of these infections becomes noticeable during epidemics, when large numbers of adults who have detectable amounts of "virus neutralizing" matter in their serum shed virus through their eliminative organs, yet do not become ill themselves.[11] What this means, apparently, is that during subclinical infections, very small amounts of virus seep through our outer immune defenses; these are so small as to not produce disease symptoms, yet are enough to stimulate immunity in healthy people.[12] This phenomenon shows that natural immunity is working, however invisible it is to us. Furthermore, it reveals that the protective dose of virus is so small that it stimulates immunity in the vast majority of people without them showing visible signs of sickness. More importantly, it demonstrates that the amount of antigen, or the aggregate amount of chemical compounds used in a vaccine, otherwise causing fevers, sore arms, malaise, convulsive seizures, allergic reactions, neurological disorders, and deaths in children, must be massive by comparison.

In addition to continuing uncertainty about the amount of antigen that is safe to use in a vaccine is the further uncertainty about what happens to vaccine antigens that remain in our bodies following immunizations. We might consider an analogy.

It is no mystery that we cannot dump raw sewage into our harbors without it having a deleterious effect on the ecosystem. It is also clear that we cannot bury oil drums or carelessly discard industrial solvents without seriously polluting the land, waters, or aquifers. Similarly, we cannot pollute our cells and blood-stream with vaccines and other toxic drugs and think that these will not produce damaging side effects over time. In the United States, following the current recommendations of the Immunization Practices Advisory Committee (1991), a baby is supposed to be immunized more than ten times before it is eighteen months old.[13] In effect, the child's bloodstream and developing immune organs are bombarded with billions of vaccine antigens and other toxic preservatives, from five or more different vaccines. Just as the insidious effect of industrial solvents does not quickly disappear from our water and land, it appears that a similar effect may be produced in our bodies by vaccines.

We have become aware that antibodies, stimulated by vac-cine antigens, are detectable in blood for years following an immunization shot. Because the detection of antibodies signals the presence of either bacterial or viral antigens, the question remains as to what eventually happens to them, especially the viral components. Because viruses are obligate parasites, they need living cells for their sustenance. The whereabouts of the untold amounts of viral antigens that are not defeated by the body's defenses following an immunization shot, shockingly, are known: vaccine antigens go inside our cells.

DNA AND VIRUSES

Viruses are parasitic non-living agents that infect living cells called host cells. Viruses invade host cells and use their enzymes to produce more viruses. Viruses consist of a nucleic acid surrounded by a protein coat. The nucleic acid DNA or RNA carries the genetic information of the cells and forms the material basis of chromosomes.[14]

Viruses are able to infect plant, animal, and bacterial cells. They also have the capacity to duplicate again and again, and during the process, often kill the host cell. Consequently, their viral offspring are released into the cellular environment where they can infect more cells.[15] Viruses can also become part of the host cells' chromosome and remain in a latent or inactive state.[16]

This condition can persist for years until some external or internal condition excites an active infection. During infection, as many as 1,000 viruses can be released in the space of one hour from one infected viral cell.[17] The problem with viruses is their behavior, i.e., the aggressive control they exert in the cellular environment. Once viral RNA or DNA becomes encoded within the infected cells' chromosomes, it is capable of duplicating like a normal gene through ongoing generations of cells.[18]

There is strong evidence that viruses, encoded in human chromosomes, may interfere with cellular processes in such a way as to produce abnormal cells, which in turn become tumors.[19] Scientists believe that cancer is an outgrowth of this infected cell process. There is also evidence that some cancers may be caused by chemicals in the environment. Cancer-causing substances, such as cigarette smoke, insecticides, and asbestos, have been found to damage DNA.[20] A certain saturation of these carcinogens, in conjunction with nutritional deficiencies and/or emotional stress, may be all that is needed to upset the dormant state of the infected cell, resulting in active infection or other disease states.

The tie-in with immunizations, as one possible cause of cancers and other chronic illness, seems more and more credible when we face the consequences of injecting large quantities of viral antigens into the body. Normally, when a virus enters the blood circulation, antibodies do not "prevent" infection per se; they "contain it."[21] Second, the presence of circulating antibodies, even in high levels, does not signify that all the viral antigens have been removed or defeated. Eventually, viruses enter a latent state within cells and are able to escape the grasp of circulating antibody. Cytomeglavirus, for example, a virus of the herpes family, can remain in body tissue for months while antibody is actively circulating in blood. There are a number of reasons for this. First, circulating antibody normally does not transverse cell membranes; this protects the invasive virus from detection.[22] Second, circulating antibody has immunosuppressive properties of its own, which constrain viral antigens within the cell.[23] This situation permits the virus to function within the host cell as a latent or inactive infection.   This condition may persist for months or even years until something—stress, worry, human catastrophe, immunosuppressive drugs, environmental pollutants, or different combinations thereof—triggers an active infection. Perhaps the latent virus presents an identity crisis for the immune system in trying to determine what this infected cell is.   This is the dilemma faced in auto-immune disorders such as acquired hemolytic anemia, rheumatic fever, rheumatoid arthritis, and lupus, in which the body directs its defense energy against itself, destroying its own cells and tissues.   It has been suggested that, during auto-immune disease, perhaps the only way the immune system can respond to these ambiguous cells is to destroy them, thereby removing "the persistence of the foreign antigenic challenge within the cells of the host."[24]

Persistent and Latent Viruses

A number of viruses have been implicated as persistent or latent, including: hepatitis B virus, herpes B viruses, and varicella-zoster type of virus. Hepatitis B virus usually occurs as an acute illness, yet it is estimated that 5 to 10 percent of people infected develop a persistent or latent virus which may linger for many years. Herpes-simplex virus type I has been implicated as a latent virus, though it is not known how the virus achieves this state within the cell.

Along with persistent and latent viruses are the related slow viruses. These viruses are characterized by extremely long incubation periods and are progressively fatal. Kuru, a degenerative condition spread by cannibalism and discovered in the 1950s among a tribe of people in New Guinea, is one such virus. Creutzfeld-Jacob disease, a slow virus disease characterized by dementia and motor convulsive disorders, is another.

It is well documented in medical literature that persistent viruses cause destruction in the form of latent or slow virus diseases or as auto-immune disorders. In these situations, it appears that a chronic condition develops, one in which host cells are either destroyed, incapacitated, or compromised in some way.   It is an antagonizing process, insidious in its destruction, that weakens the entire immune system, draining it slowly from the inside out.   As the immune system grows weaker, its ability to protect us from other infections is greatly impaired.   If this is true, then childhood immunizations, having released billions of bacterial and viral antigens into our body and consequently into our cells, may have progressively debilitated the natural immunity of generation upon generation of children for the last 200 years.   It seems not only possible but highly probable that immunizations have planted the seeds of infections and chronic disease states.

CHAPTER 4

The Making of a Vaccine

So far, we have observed vaccines as being foreign to the immune system, without fully defining the scope of their being foreign. The composition of a vaccine is much more than a simple bacterial or viral antigen. Any discussion of vaccines, either as foreign protein elements or as probable causes of persistent infections, allergic reactions, or systemic illness, would not be complete without investigating the different types of vaccines and how they are produced.

LIVE AND KILLED VACCINES

Before we see how a vaccine is produced in the laboratory, it would be helpful to define the different types of vaccines that are administered to infants and children. In general, there are two major types: those that are made from bacteria and those that are made from viruses. Vaccines are further distinguished as being either live or killed preparations.

Before a live vaccine can become suitable for human use, it has to be weakened or attenuated, so as not to cause disease in its recipients. There are several methods of attenuating a live virus. Perhaps the most relied upon yet bizarre way is by serial passage. During serial passage a virus strain is passed through animal cells a number of times. It is not uncommon for some viruses to be propagated fifty times or more to reduce their potency. During vaccine production, measles virus is passed through chick embryo cells, polio virus through monkey kidney cells, rubella virus through duck or rabbit cells, and yellow fever virus through mice and chick embryo.[1]

Killed vaccines are extracts that are inactivated by the use of radiation, heat, or chemicals. The immunizing particles of a killed vaccine are derived from the disease agent in the vaccine and may be whole cells, split organisms that are chemically extracted, synthesized molecules, or toxoids.[2] The influenza vaccine, the hepatitis B vaccine, and the Salk polio vaccine are all examples of killed preparations. The essential difference between a "live" vaccine and a "killed" one is that the "live" antigen can reproduce in the person receiving the vaccine, while the killed one does not.[3] However clearcut this distinction looks, there have been serious problems with killed vaccines which defy their inability to reproduce in their recipients.

The primary response in the body to a killed vaccine is the production of circulating antibodies. While the importance of circulating antibodies is undeniable, the role of circulating antibodies is primarily in preventing disease, not in preventing infection from occurring. Infection can—and does—occur after the administration of a killed vaccine, although, in theory, it is confined to the person receiving the vaccine.

It was thus thought that mass vaccination programs with killed vaccines would inhibit the spread of infection and disease. However, this belief was proven faulty by a number of vaccine disasters that could be traced to some aspect of vaccine production, in which infective virus still remained in the vaccine culture or failed to be inactivated properly. In 1955, for example, after the administration of the Salk polio vaccine on a mass scale, a clustering of paralytic polio cases occurred not only in recently vaccinated children but also in family and community contacts. Formalin, the germicide that was used to inactivate the polio virus, was found to be the cause of the mishap, as it failed to inactivate all the batches of polio virus.

VIRUS VACCINES

The two childhood vaccines that are constituted from viruses are the MMR vaccine and the polio vaccine. The MMR vaccine is a killed virus preparation that combines the measles, mumps, and rubella antigens into a single vaccine. The polio vaccine comes in two varieties, the killed virus and the live virus. The oral polio vaccine, which is the live (attenuated) vaccine, is presently used to immunize school children. It became available in 1961 and eventually replaced the Salk vaccine as the preferred vaccine for children.

The live polio vaccine combines three different strains of polio virus, which are grown in monkey kidney cells or in human diploid cells. They are propagated in the presence of a nutrient broth consisting of dextrose, sodium bicarbonate, antibiotics (neomycin or streptomycin), amino acids, phenol red (a PH indicator), and calf serum.[4] The final product is diluted, and sorbitol is added as a stabilizer.[5]

The killed polio virus is produced in a similar way, except that the virus is inactivated with formaldehyde. Other viral vaccines such as measles, mumps, influenza, and yellow fever are cultivated in chick and duck embryos.[6]

BACTERIAL VACCINES

The primary vaccine that is made from bacteria is diphtheria. During the early 1900s, two distinct diphtheria vaccines were used on a limited scale: diphtheria antiserum and diphtheria toxin-antitoxin mixture (TAM). The alleged protection from antiserum came from antibodies that were produced in the blood of horses (after the animals were deliberately inoculated with diphtheria organisms and later bled) for the distinct purpose of making a protective serum for humans. The antiserum was used by those people lacking a predetermined level of circulating antitoxin (natural antidote) in their own blood to diphtheria as determined by the Schick test, usually in lieu of being exposed to diphtheria or immediately after being exposed to the disease. A second diphtheria vaccine (TAM) was used for active immunization and was available for all those who wished to experience science rather than taking their chances with nature and their own natural immunity to diphtheria. Even with the antitoxin component in the vaccine, toxin and antidote combined, the vaccine was considered too dangerous for human use and many vaccine accidents occurred.[7] Scientists responded by developing a new diphtheria vaccine prepared from toxoids. Toxoids are toxins that have been rendered nonpoisonous by the use of a chemical agent. In the 1920s, when diphtheria toxoids were being developed, formalin (formaldehyde) was chosen as the chemical disinfectant of choice.

DPT: Manufacture and Ingredients

The preparation of the DPT vaccine combines the toxoids of diphtheria and tetanus with the whole cells of pertussis bacteria to form a single vaccine. During the first stage of production, large amounts of tetanus and diphtheria are grown in a broth. Toxins are the poisonous materials synthesized by the tetanus and diphtheria organisms. Tetanus toxins are produced in a culture broth of dextrose, beef heart infusion, sodium chloride, and casein.[8] Diphtheria toxin is produced in a similar culture. After the required amount of toxin is produced, the culture is filtered. Formalin is added to the rich toxin broth and the culture is maintained at the most favorable temperature for two or three weeks.[9] However, further purification of the toxoids is still necessary because of the many impurities still left in the mixture. One way this is accomplished is through a process called alcohol fractionation, in which methanol is employed to precipitate the toxoid. As a result the toxoid becomes a powder and is then "dissolved" in a buffer that contains glycine.[10] It is then further sterilized.

The killed whole cells of pertussis bacteria are the final component of the DPT vaccine. The organisms are grown in a medium of hydrolysate of casein, minerals, and other materials.[11] The bacteria are killed and detoxified by heat or by adding the anti-infective chemical thimerosal to the mixture.[12] Finally, an adjuvant (antibody-boosting substance) such as aluminum hydroxide or aluminum potassium sulfate is added.[13] The final DPT product combines the diphtheria and tetanus toxoids with the killed whole cells of the pertussis bacteria.

FDA TESTS FOR DPT VACCINE

Childhood vaccines are tested on mice and guinea pigs to determine potency and safety requirements for humans. Laboratory tests are carried out by the Division of Biologic Standards, a part of the Public Health Service. In 1948, the safety test for the DPT vaccine became more stringent after Randolph Byers and Frederick Moll of Harvard Medical School validated that severe neurological disorders followed the administration of DPT vaccine.[14] Their research was performed at Children's Hospital in Boston and was published in *Pediatrics* in 1948. Although their findings shocked the medical community, nothing was done by physicians to halt the use of the DPT vaccine. As of 1992, some forty-four years after their research, the vaccine is still being used to immunize our infants.

Potency Test

The potency test for the DPT vaccine involves a two-part experiment. In general, a highest and lowest immunizing potency are established by testing different dilutions of the vaccine on separate groups of mice. First, mice are vaccinated with a test dose of pertussis vaccine. A second inoculation, called a challenge dose, is injected into the same mice fourteen to seventeen days later.[15] This is done to establish the effectiveness of the test dose. However, before the challenge dose is introduced, 87.5 percent of the mice must have survived the test dose.[16] A segment of the potency test for the DPT vaccine is described in the *Federal Register*.

> The mice shall be observed for 14 days. Mice dying within 72 hours after challenge shall be excluded from the test. Records shall be maintained of the number of mice showing both paralysis and enlargement of the head at the end of 14 days. All mice that show both paralysis and enlargenent shall be considered as deaths for the purposes of determining the ED 50.[17]

In what appears to be a mathematical formula, an estimate of vaccine potency is extrapolated from the mouse tests and applied to humans. The FDA sheds more light on this process:

> The number of protective units of the total human immunizing dose shall be estimated for each lot of vaccine from the results of simultaneous intercerebral mouse protection tests of the vaccine under test and the U.S. Standard Pertussis Vaccine.[18]

Safety Test

The trial for vaccine safety is known as the mouse toxicity test. During this procedure, the pertussis vaccine is injected into the abdominal cavities of the mice. The main criterion for vaccine safety is determined by how much or how little weight the mice gain or lose over two allotted time periods: seventy-two hours and seven days.[19] Another safety factor is that no more that 5 percent of the mice may die after the seven day period.[20] The results of these tests, and perhaps other factors, determine whether the vaccine makes it to the marketplace.

In general, these are the methods by which the final DPT vaccine antigen levels are deemed acceptable and safe for our children. Charles Manclark, a Food and Drug Administration specialist, remarked in 1976, that "the DPT vaccine had one of the worst failure rates of any product submitted to the Bureau of Biologics for testing."[21] After some forty-five years of testing for safety and potency, children are still suffering side effects and severe neurological disorders from the DPT vaccine.

CHAPTER 5

Vaccination and
Animal Experimentation

*T*he production of vaccines is directly related to experimentation on animals. Each year thousands of rabbits, mice, hamsters, rats, guinea pigs, pigs, horses, sheep, and donkeys are bled so that their antibodies can be used in the production of antiserums.[1] Since the 1950s, hundreds of thousands of rhesus monkeys and green monkeys have been sacrificed so that polio vaccine could be grown in their kidney cells. The brain tissue of horses, sheep, and dogs has been used for many years to prepare rabies vaccines.[2] Rabbits, dogs, ducks, chickens, and guinea pigs are sacrificed to make cell cultures for live rubella and measles vaccines.[3] In the small country of Holland, whose figures on animal experimentation are available, there were 1,208,539 animals used in medical research in 1986, of which 21 percent or 250,950 were experimented on for biological products: vaccines, serums, and other blood products.[4] It has been conservatively estimated that if about 10 percent of all the animals used in animal research worldwide are employed in some aspect of vaccine production, then ten to twenty million animals are maimed or sacrificed each year to produce vaccines, serums, and other blood products.

The courageous work of animal rights activists has called attention to the inhuman and sometimes barbaric treatment animals are forced to endure in military, other government, corporate, and university laboratories.

The Draize Test

The Draize test is a cruel method of chemical testing, employed by the Food and Drug Administration and by some

31

chemical companies, that measures the amount of eye irritation and skin damage caused by cosmetics. During the test strong concentrations of cosmetic chemicals are "dripped" into rabbits' eyes.[5] Afterwards researchers measure the effects of the injuries produced by the intense burning. Redness and swelling are common reactions, and in severe cases, a total loss of vision occurs.[6] Naturally, rabbits try to shut their eyes or use their paws to remove the irritating substances. Researchers have found a way to prevent the rabbits from doing this, so as to not interfere with their own test results. To control the rabbits' natural impulse they use mechanical holding devices which immobilize the rabbits' bodies in place with only their heads sticking out.[7] Next, they fasten metal clips to the rabbits' eyelids to keep them open.[8] Now the rabbits have no protection against the wicked perversions of the laboratory workers and must endure this senseless torture without defense. This is just one of many experiments that are performed on animals in the name of scientific research.

More Experimentations

In 1961 the Atomic Energy Commission financed experiments with radioactive chemicals. In one experiment carried out at the Lovelace Foundation in Albuquerque, New Mexico, sixty-four dogs were forced to inhale radioactive strontium 90 as part of a larger experiment that compared the effects of injected strontium 90 with the inhaled chemical. Twenty-five beagles died as a result of inhaling strontium 90.[9]

At the University of Rochester School of Medicine more beagles were put through such rigors in the name of scientific advancement. In this experiment fifty dogs were confined to crates and then doused with x-ray radiation.[10] The aim of the experiment was to determine what dosage of radiation would kill 50 percent of the animals. (This test called the LD50 is commonly used by the government and private industry to test new drugs and vaccines.) As a result of the radiation, twenty-one of the dogs died between the ninth and the thirty-ninth day following irradiation, many from internal hemorrhaging.[11]

The prestigious magazine, *Science,* has presented a number of articles over the years describing animal experimentations. An article entitled "Chronic Uncontrolled Cross-Circulation in Unanesthetized Dogs," published in 1955, is particularly noteworthy. During the animal experiments discussed, which were carried out at the Naval Medical Research Institute in Bethesda, Maryland, two dogs were joined together at the neck with polyethylene tubing connecting one dog's neck artery to the other's jugular vein.[12] The necks of the two dogs were then wrapped together and held in place with a plaster cast, forcing the animals' heads to tilt back—and stay back in place. The animals were forced to endure this treatment for seventy-two hours. This demented experiment demonstrated that blood could successfully cross-circulate from one animal to another for extended periods of time.

These are just a few of the medical experiments, chosen from among scores, that are performed on animals each year in the name of scientific advancement. Because the production of vaccines also involves the sacrificing of thousands of animals each year, descriptions of how polio and smallpox vaccine were made in years past are included. Although the descriptions which follow are circa 1900 for smallpox vaccine and 1952 for polio vaccine, they are far from being outdated. The chemicals that are used in vaccine production change from decade to decade, yet the change is of little significance. After 192 years of vaccine production, scientists still cannot make a safe vaccine.

THE MAKING OF POLIO VACCINE IN 1952

In years preceding the arrival of Jonas Salk's polio vaccine in 1955, experiments were performed in laboratories to determine the correct dose of antigen and supplementary chemicals to use in the polio vaccine. One of the first steps in preparing the vaccine was to create a suitable culture for the virus to grow in. During the making of polio vaccine in 1952, Hanks' balanced salt solution was used. Added to this were phenol red, a chemical used as an indicator of virus-antibody activity, and chloroform, a highly-toxic chemical once used in anesthesia, but here probably used as a preservative.[13] Other separate components of the final culture medium consisted of: horse serum, ox serum, chicken plasma, and chicken embryo extract.[14] The chicken extract was made by combining the entire "nine-day old" gestating chickens, including their heads and their eyes, adding Hanks' salt solution, and grinding the mixture in a blender.[15] It was then centrifuged, frozen, thawed, frozen again, and stored for future use. The final culture consisted of varying percentages of horse serum or ox serum, Hanks' salt solution, and chicken embryo extract. Finally, the antibiotics penicillin and streptomycin were added to the swilling caldron.[16]

The next step in the process is to add animal or human tissue to the culture so that the polio virus has a suitable environment in which to grow. In these experiments, the tissue was derived from the testes of rhesus monkeys. After the testes were surgically removed, they were cut into little pieces with scissors and placed into test tubes where they came in contact with the culture medium.[17] This tissue culture was incubated for a number of days, after which the fluid was drained from the mixture. Finally, the three different strains of polio virus were introduced into the tissue culture, where they remained for a short period of time. Fresh culture was then added and the entire mixture subsequently incubated.[18]

There were three types of polio virus used to make the vaccine: the Mahoney, Lansing, and Saukett strains. The source of the Mahoney virus was "suspensions" of spinal cord from paralyzed monkeys.[19] The material was attenuated by passing the virus through the monkeys' cells nine times. The Lansing virus was a suspension of mouse spinal cord and brain that had passed through the mice or mice cells eighteen times. A second component of the Lansing strain was a "subculture" of virus in human tissue. The Lansing virus was provided by John Enders who, along with his colleagues Weller and Robbins of Harvard, in 1949, propagated polio virus in human foreskin.[20] The last strain, or the Saukett virus, was procured directly from human feces.[21]

PROBLEMS WITH VACCINES USING ANIMAL CELLS

The serial passage of virus through animals or animal cells is necessary—by definition—to reduce the virulence of the vaccine virus. It is one of the ways viral vaccines are attenuated or weakened for human use. However, the serial passage of virus can become fatal to nerve tissue (neurovirulent) during animal passage and has become so after being injected into man.[22] During the 1940s a catastrophe of this sort occurred in French West Africa during a large yellow fever immunization campaign. During vaccine production the yellow fever virus was propagated in mouse brain 258 times.[23] The last two animal passages produced the sought-after strain. The laboratory mice who became paralyzed as a result were subsequently killed and their brains removed. In what sounds like a true horror story, the mouse brains were pulverized and then freeze-dried.[24] The mouse brain/yellow fever virus was used by the French to immunize thousands of Africans in French West Africa in 1944. As a result, there were 102 reported cases of meningoencephalitis and 18 deaths among the 102,000 vaccinees.[25]

The production of live viruses has brought to the forefront the enormous difficulties of producing uncontaminated vaccine products. The vaccine virus culture can become contaminated from "extraneous" substances or from more deadly strains of virus in the laboratory, especially if production and research workers interact without using extreme caution.[26] One serious problem has been the occurrence of actively poisonous virus strains that have found their way unnoticed into the final vaccine, which nevertheless has been administered to humans. Undoubtedly, the most serious untoward effect of vaccine production is the contamination of virus originating from the material the virus is grown in: animal cells, animal serum, and human serum. During the 1950s, tens of millions of doses of polio vaccine were produced from virus grown in infected monkey kidney cells. Since the late 1950s, many of these "simian viruses" had been isolated by scientists and were discovered to be contaminating polio vaccines. One such simian virus, named SV40, found in both Salk and Sabin polio virus, is resistant to the neutralizing effects of formalin, yet nevertheless was passed on to unsuspecting millions of people who received the polio vaccine in the 1950s and early 1960s.[27]

Many of the live viruses that are used to propagate vaccine cultures such as polio, yellow fever, measles, mumps, and rubella organisms are grown in chicken, duck, and rabbit embryo. It has been shown that chicken eggs are susceptible to an entire spectrum of avian (bird-related) viruses, which can be transferred to humans through the vaccine.[28] Secondly, living vaccines that are produced from human serums have caused dangerous occurrences of hepatitis in the population because of the hepatitis B virus that is present in some of the serum.[29] Two other substances used in vaccine production that have been identified as possible sources of viral contamination are tryspin (used to disperse cells) and animal serum (used as a medium in cell growth). They are thought to be "possible sources" of contamination from mycoplasma, bacteriophages, reoviruses, and parvoviruses.[30]

The apparent danger of using animal serums foreign to man and animal serums foreign to other animals has been known for hundreds of years and was reported in medical literature as early as 1667 when lambs' blood was tried unsuccessfully for a human blood transfusion.[31] It was quickly discovered to be a precarious endeavor, and the practice was soon abandoned, at least for a while. Regardless, however, the practice of using animal proteins in vaccines and serums has had a long history of use— with disastrous results.

Serum sickness is the name given to a condition caused by an allergic reaction to a foreign animal protein, and in the case of diphtheria antiserum, a reaction to horse blood, the strange and nauseating material used to concoct the antidote to diphtheria. Serum sickness is characterized by fever, edema (excessive accumulation of fluid in the tissues), swelling of the lymphatic glands, and a uticarial (extremely itchy) rash which envelops the entire body.[32] Other symptoms such as joint pain and bloody diarrhea, though less common, may also be present. Medical literature is filled with reports of minor to severe allergic reactions following the use of diphtheria, tetanus, scarlet fever, and plague vaccines. In 1896 Gottstein reported that serum sickness brought on by diphtheria antitoxin occurred in 23 percent of the cases he investigated.[33] In 1909 Weaver revealed that a rash occurred in 56 percent of people receiving either diphtheria or plague antiserum.[34] In 1942, Ferdinand Kojis, a practicing physician at the Willard Park Hospital in New York, reported that 11 percent of his patients suffered serum sickness after receiving injections of scarlet fever or diphtheria antiserums.[35]

SMALLPOX VACCINE

The nature of the materials found in vaccines is both disgusting and grotesque. Yet no vaccine was more unsightly than smallpox vaccine. The method in which smallpox vaccine was procured from the cow at the turn of the century, and continuing well into the twentieth century, is perhaps the most loathsome practice of all. The following is a description (summarized from a number of sources) outlining how smallpox vaccine was produced dating from the early 1900s.

A young calf, usually about three months old, is strapped down securely to an operating table. An area of about 15 inches square is shaved from the calf's stomach or abdomen. Between thirty to fifty inch-long incisions are made into the animal's stomach with a sharp lancet. Smallpox lymph and glycerine are then rubbed into each cut. After this procedure, the animal is returned to a holding stable and positioned in such a way so that it will be unable to lick its sores, thus inibiting the animal's natural instinct to take care of itself. In a matter of hours, or days, the calf becomes very sick with fever. Shortly thereafter, smallpox vesicles appear on the calf's skin, scabs form, and the processes of eliminating impurities from the blood begin. After about six days the smallpox scabs become filled with a gross mass of fluid and pus underneath and the calf is once again strapped to the operating table. The area around the incisions is washed with warm water and each protruding smallpox vesicle is secured with a clamp. The smallpox crust is then scraped from each sore with a blunt lancet, and the remaining contents of blood, skin, lymph, and pus are drawn from each sore and transferred to a heat-resistant pot. Glycerine is added to the poisonous swill, and the entire contents are mixed with an electric motor. They are then passed through a sieve to remove the coarse materials (rotten flesh, hair etc.) and homogenized again by remixing the witch's brew. The mixture is then poured into tubes and sold throughout the country as pure calf lymph, commonly known as smallpox vaccine.[36-38]

This is what smallpox vaccine really is. This is the material that was injected into millions of children and adults from about 1880 to 1940. This vile material was supposed to prevent someone from getting smallpox!

Historically, horse blood, sheep blood, monkey and rabbit kidney tissue, chicken embryo, mouse brain, dog brain, duck cells, and calf serum have all been used to produce antibodies or to grow vaccine cell cultures that eventually find their way into the bodies of millions of children and adults.

The production of laboratory virus at the turn of the century and during the 1940s and 1950s gives us a much clearer picture of what was never openly revealed to the American public, a description of the materials used in vaccine production. The materials were so toxic, gross, and nauseating to contemplate, that any person would question their use, simply out of common sense. What any of these noxious materials had to do with preventing disease in children or how any scientist-physician could consider combining these gross materials in a vaccine vial, regardless of dosage amounts, and inject them into the delicate arms of millions of infants and children, is beyond comprehension.

CHAPTER 6

Witch's Brew:
Toxic Chemicals in Vaccines

A ny discussion of vaccines, either as foreign elements or as probable causes of persistent infections, would not be complete without an investigation of some of the chemicals used in their production and the possible role they might play in initiating allergic, systemic, or neurological damage in children.

Many of the chemicals that are used in vaccine production are largely unknown to the general public—even to many medical practitioners. Some of these chemicals are extremely toxic and are known carcinogens (cancer-causing agents). In this chapter we will explore three chemicals that are routinely used in vaccine production: thimerosal (mercury-preservative), aluminum sulfate (vaccine adjuvant), and formalin (a germicide).

One of the problems that I faced was to determine if the amount of hazardous substances found in vaccines was contributing to a wide range of adverse reactions suffered by infants and children. Of equal importance was the possibility that the combination of mercury, aluminum, and formaldehyde (along with many other chemicals in the vaccine, including vaccine antigens), might have created a kind of time bomb whose ultimate outcome was being played out in the cells, tissues, and blood of the human body, and whose effect no scientist would venture to predict. Equally important was the cumulative effect these chemicals might have on a baby, since all healthy infants are scheduled to be immunized ten to twelve times before they're eighteen months old!

The problem became more difficult to approach when I discovered that there was very little written about the role of mercury, aluminum, and formaldehyde (and other immunizing chemicals) in producing adverse vaccine reactions. While drug companies openly acknowledge in their package inserts that thimerosal, egg protein, and streptomycin-neomycin are three substances in a vaccine to which infants and children may be allergic, I found only one article in a medical journal that reported vigorous tests of vaccine chemicals for their carcinogenic potential. Even though the chemicals produced tumors in test animals, there was not even a hint that they posed any real health threat to infants and children receiving them in the form of a vaccine. I suspect that the lack of articles on this subject is due to the perception that the amounts of these substances in vaccines are far too small to cause any real damage to infants. I vehemently disagree.

There is no lack of material in the medical literature, however, on the toxic effects of mercury, aluminum, and formaldehyde. Therefore, many of the adverse reactions to these chemicals that this chapter discusses derive from studies of a wide range of applications; many are unrelated, as such, to vaccinations. Moreover, the amount of toxic substance that caused the adverse reaction is probably a lot higher than the amounts found in a .5 ml. dose of vaccine. However, with any toxic substance, no one knows for sure what exact amount, large or small, will initiate an allergic or systemic reaction or perhaps a more serious chronic internal injury. What used to be an acceptable limit for a noxious substance many years ago is invariably lowered many times as new discoveries are made and more accidents occur. When you're dealing with poisonous material whose ultimate effect on the human organism can only be viewed as detrimental, the amounts that are considered hazardous are always somewhat arbitrary—very little is written in stone. With all of this in mind, I suspect that the mercury, aluminum, formaldehyde, and other noxious agents used in vaccine production are not only initiating allergic reactions in infants and children, but are also a contributing factor toward more serious adverse vaccine reactions.

THIMEROSAL

During the 1920s, many new chemicals were tested for their ability to destroy microorganisms. The collective name antimicrobials was given to describe these chemicals, which were often used as germicides or antiseptics. One germicide that came under evaluation during this period was ethyl mercuri thiosalicylic acid, an organic mercury compound, known as merthiolate. It is now more commonly referred to as thimerosal and is used extensively in vaccines as a preservative.

Early Experiments

In 1930 Powell and Jamieson tested thimerosal for its ability to inhibit huge cultures of bacteria and yeast.[1] A solution of 1 percent thimerosal, concentrated at 1:10,000, was able to kill large cultures of streptococci and pneumococci without destroying the bacterial antigen.[2] This was significant because the antigen in a vaccine is the agent that stimulates immunity and therefore should theoretically never be destroyed. Thimerosal was even able to sterilize culture plates, eliminating microorganisms in one to five days at 20° centigrade.[3] When the germicide was diluted in serum globulin, it killed staphylococcus aureus germs after twenty-four hours.[4]

Animal Tests

Powell and Jamieson injected varying amounts of thimerosal into rats, guinea pigs, dogs, and rabbits, to determine the toxicity of the germicide. The "tolerated" dose for rabbits was 25 milligrams per kilogram of body weight.[5] Of the forty-one rabbits tested, twenty-nine rabbits lived (71 percent) and twelve died (29 percent). When the dosage was increased, just 10 milligrams, only four rabbits lived (15 percent) while twenty-two (85 percent) died of poisoning effects.[6] When thimerosal was injected into the abdominal wall of guinea pigs, the animals experienced great pain. Their hair became erect, their abdomens rigid, and their backs arched.[7]

Human Tests

Each member of a group of twenty-two people ranging in age from two to fifty-four years old received a dose of 1 percent thimerosal in the amount of 50 cc (some also receiving a second dose), to test the safety of the chemical.[8] Afterwards, one case of nephritis and another of thrombophlebitis were observed. However, according to the attending physician, the germicide did not prove to be toxic to its recipients and did not produce "shock symptoms." There was no mention in the study of any qualifying tests being performed (blood, urine) which may have established the chemical's effect on human cells and tissue or how much mercury was retained in the body. It appears that the final evaluation of thimerosal, regarding its safe or unsafe use in human beings, was made solely by observation. I find that disturbing, especially in light of the attending physician's concluding remarks which were, "the beneficial effect of the drug was not definitely proven...."[9] While the results of these early tests proved that thimerosal was able to kill bacteria in vitro (test tubes) Powell and Jamieson, the authors of the article, concluded that the germicide may still be destructive to tissue.[10]

A Poor Antiseptic

During the 1930s and 1940s, new revelations about thimerosal and its ability to kill microorganisms, especially in the presence of human serum and other body fluids, began to cast a dark shadow on this once highly regarded antiseptic. In 1948 the disinfectant properties of thimerosal and two other organomercurial compounds were reviewed in a study conducted by Harry Morton, Frank Engley, and Leon North.[11] When thimerosal was mixed in a culture broth of beef extract and horse serum, it failed to kill hemolytic streptococci after an exposure time of ten minutes.[12] More importantly, when the germicide-culture was injected into the test mice, sixteen of seventeen mice died.[13] The authors concluded that thimerosal was not effective, either as a germicide or as an antiseptic, because the bacteria with which it came into contact were still able to cause infection, even death.

Thimerosal is described in medical literature as having a strong bacteriostatic action (arresting bacterial growth), yet having a slow bactericidal effect (destroying the organism). In 1950, Philip Price confirmed the dual properties of thimerosal. It became bactericidal when it came into contact with disease organisms for progressively longer periods of time. In his experiments, thimerosal, in a concentration of 1:50,000 and in solution with a neutralizing agent, killed only 3 percent of colon bacilli after one minute of exposure. However, after two hours of exposure, it killed 99 percent of the bacilli.[14] Conversely, diluted thimerosal without the neutralizing solution killed 96 percent of E. coli bacteria in one minute.[15] It appears that even when microorganisms are exposed to thimerosal for a short amount of time, some will be destroyed and others merely inhibited.

Early tests demonstrated that thimerosal could kill large numbers of bacteria and that it held great promise as an effective germicide. Later tests seemed to prove the opposite: that it had a limited ability to kill pathogenic bacteria and so was a poor antiseptic. Further experiments revealed that it randomly killed or inhibited bacterial growth without any selectivity. Applying these observations to vaccines, it would appear that thimerosal cannot be depended on to do the impossible: to selectively prevent the growth of extraneous, unwanted bacteria and yet not harm the bacterial or viral antigens in the vaccine. If this is true, then thimerosal may alter the potency of vaccines, in some cases, rendering them completely inactive.

Thimerosal Destroys Vaccine Potency

This matter was put to the test in the 1950s, at the suggestion of Dr. Jonas Salk, a man whose name has become synonymous with the inactivated polio vaccine. In a personal communication to researcher Edwin Davisson, Salk commented that thimerosal adversely affected the potency of his polio vaccine, especially when the vaccine was subjected to heat during incubation and when the vaccine was being shipped during the hot summer months.[16] During heat stability experiments, thimerosal, in a concentration of 1:10,000, caused "severe damage" to the type 1 polio virus after five days of incubation at 37° centigrade.[17] The type 2 polio virus preserved in the same concentration became completely impotent after ten days of heating at the same temperature.[18] These tests confirmed what Salk had suspected: namely, that when thimerosal was used as a preservative for polio vaccine, it severely altered the vaccine's potency. During the experiments, a secondary, unanticipated complication ensued: the presence of residual heavy metal, namely copper, in the final vaccine. It was shown that this metal could influence the deterioration of thimerosal by oxidation. In order to remedy this situation and to solve the problem of polio antigen deterioration caused by thimerosal, still another preservative, EDTA, had to be added to the vaccine culture. In order to stabilize the vaccine, twenty-five times the normal amount of EDTA had to be added.[19]

The presence of thimerosal, used as a preservative in vaccines and immune serums, has been shown to be very inadequate. Its success as a germicide seems to be tied to how long the germicide remains in contact with the vaccine culture. If extraneous bacteria or viruses in the vaccine, some highly pathogenic, are merely inhibited by thimerosal and not killed, will those organisms be harmful after the vaccine is injected into human tissue and blood? Second, if the potency of the vaccine is destroyed by thimerosal, what exactly is this serum in the vaccine vial? And third, if thimerosal can kill some bacterial cells and inhibit the growth or multiplication of others, what effect will it have on healthy human cells after the vaccine serum is injected into our bloodstream? The answer to this last disturbing question is perhaps the most crucial—and is at least more readily available.

Thimerosal Inhibits the Action of White Blood Cells

In 1937, Salle created a toxicity index for germicides. He tested nine different germicides and discovered that mercurochrome and thimerosal had the highest toxicity for body tissue.[20] In 1940, Welch and Hunter, adopting Salle's toxicity index, studied the effects of germicides on phagocytosis, a crucial immune function occurring in animals and humans in which white blood cells called leukocytes ingest foreign microorganisms, thereby protecting host cells from invaders. In earlier experiments performed in 1928, Alexander Fleming had demonstrated that when leukocytes were filtered from the blood, blood lost its bactericidal power.[21]

One of the experiments performed by Welch and Hunter was to test germicides for their ability to prevent or inhibit phagocytosis. Two commonly used germicide/ disinfectants used to preserve vaccines, antiserums, and plasmas were tested: phenol and thimerosal. To determine the effects of the germicides on the phagocytosis of staphylococci, the germicides were mixed individually with cultures of guinea pig blood and human blood until a certain dilution of the germicide stopped the action of phagocytosis.[22] Phenol completely inhibited phagocytosis in guinea pig blood and human blood in concentrations of 1:500 and 1:400 respectively.[23] Thimerosal completely prevented phagocytosis in guinea pig blood and human blood in concentrations of 1:24,000 and 1:17,000 respectively.[24]

Thimerosal is commonly used as an antiseptic/preservative in vaccines in the range of 1:10,000 to 1:20,000. Welch's and Hunter's 1940 findings, applied to current thimerosal use in vaccines, lead to the conclusion that thimerosal completely inhibits phagocytosis in blood, one of the body's most vital immune defenses!

As a final point, a toxicity index was drawn up based on Salle's model. Welch and Hunter established that phenol and thimerosal were 4 and 5.7 times more toxic for human cells than for the staphylococci germs.[25] Mercurochrome, a popular household mercurial antiseptic used during the 1950s and 1960s, was 29.3 times more toxic for human cells than it was for the bacteria.[26]

Thimerosal in Serum

Thimerosal is also used as a preservative in serum, blood plasma, and gamma globulin. In 1935, Salle and Lazarus demonstrated that thimerosal was thirty-five times more toxic for "embryonic tissue cells than for staphylococcus aureus."[27] In 1939, Nye and Welch reported that thimerosal was more toxic for leukocytes (white blood cells) than for bacterial cells.[28] Other researchers arrived at similar conclusions. In 1942, Johnson and Meleney found that thimerosal worked poorly in checking blood contamination in plasma.[29] In 1944, Waller discovered that thimerosal destroyed the anti-Rh agglutinins in anti-Rh serum.[30] In 1948, Morton and associates reported that thimerosal did not have strong antiseptic abilities, especially when mixed in serums or other mediums containing protein.[31]

Mercury Poisoning

A study published in the *British Medical Journal* in 1979 revealed that nineteen of twenty-six patients (73 percent) receiving immunoglobulin serum preserved with thimerosal had "raised" mercury levels in their body, qualified by urine analysis. The authors concluded that patients receiving long-term therapy of this kind were "theoretically" at risk from the mercury in thimerosal.[32] In 1969, Suzuki reported a case of acute thimerosal poisoning in a thirteen-year-old boy suffering from intestinal disease. He had been receiving plasma over a three-month period.[33]

Pink disease (acrodynia) is a condition characterized by restlessness, sensitivity to light (photophobia), and general misery, in which the outer extremities become painful, swollen, and red. Thousands of infants suffered from pink disease between 1890 and 1950, caused by the mercury (mercurous chloride) in teething powders. Those products are now prohibited. In 1980 a case of acrodynia was reported in a twenty-year-old male suffering from congenital agammaglobulinemia. His gamma globulin preparation was preserved with thimerosal and he had been receiving the treatment for about fifteen years.[34]

The author's conclusion was that people who receive regular injections of gamma globulin are potentially at risk from the mercury in thimerosal.

Allergic Reactions

Probably the best-known reaction to mercury compounds is in the form of allergic reactions. In 1944 Hollander reported a case of contact dermatitis caused by thimerosal.[35] Allergic contact dermatitis occurs when an individual becomes sensitized to an allergen during an "induction" period usually lasting between ten to twenty-one days.[36] After the cycle of sensitization is completed, allergic reactions can occur if the allergen is reintroduced. Reactions can persist for months or occur over a lifetime. Other factors such as the type of chemical, its concentration, and the length of exposure all play a part in whether an allergic reaction will be elicited.[37]

Diagnostic patch testing is the vehicle used to measure allergic reactions in a sensitized group. A small amount of allergen, proven to be non-irritating in a control group, is applied to the skin of members of the sensitized group. Readings of allergic reactions are then made. In 1973 Rudner reported the results of diagnostic patch testing conducted by the North American Contact Dermatitis Group and the International Contact Dermatitis Group. Of ten common allergens tested, three were chemicals routinely found in vaccines: thimerosal, neomycin (an antibiotic), and formalin. Thimerosal produced positive allergic reactions in 8 percent of the people tested; formalin in 6 percent of the test group, and neomycin in 4 percent.[38]

ALUMINUM

One of the first cases of aluminum poisoning was reported by Spofforth in 1921. Betts described the health hazards of aluminum in drinking water and in medicines as early as 1926.[39] Despite the wisdom of these initial cautionary findings, their warnings were not heeded. Until the 1960s, nearly all the reports of health risks and accidents associated with aluminum focused on factory workers and the dangers they faced from inhaling dust particles at aluminum production plants. Since that time, however, aluminum toxicity has been reported in many other areas of health.

Aluminum poisoning has been confirmed as a source of contamination in people receiving long-term dialysis treatment for renal (kidney) failure. Aluminum salts or aluminum hydroxide gels are given orally to patients suffering from renal failure for the management of excessive phosphates which often accompany this chronic kidney condition. Ordinary tap water has been cited as a source of aluminum and also as a source of aluminum poisoning in hemodialysis patients, as water is a key component of dialysis therapy. There is also evidence that aluminum in tap water or from gels accumulates in the tissues of people receiving hemodialysis. In animal studies, when "modest" oral and injected doses of aluminum salts were fed to rats suffering from the toxic effects of excess urea in their blood (and also fed to those who did not), it produced, in both groups, a significant amount of aluminum in the liver, serum, heart, brain, and bone tissue, resulting in lethargy, anorexia, bleeding, and finally death.[40] In human studies, excessive aluminum has been discovered in hemodialysis patients suffering from chronic renal failure. The absorbed aluminum was found in excess in tissues and serum.[41]

The accumulation of aluminum found in people receiving long-term dialysis therapy has been described as a severe neurological syndrome, known as dialysis encephalopathy. In 1972 Alfrey and colleagues described this disease as manifesting symptoms such as speech disorders, dementia, and convulsions.[42] According to their research, the underlying cause was an increased amount of aluminum in the brain, muscle, and bone tissue. In 1976 Burks and associates demonstrated that this brain condition was the chief cause of death in one dialysis treatment center.[43] In 1983 Griswold and fellow researchers showed that children who suffered renal failure and were not receiving dialysis treatment, but were taking aluminum hydroxide orally, also suffered from encephalopathy.[44] All these research findings strongly suggest that aluminum is neurotoxic.

ALUMINUM AND OIL ADJUVANTS IN VACCINES

An adjuvant is a chemical agent that is added to a drug to enhance its effect. Adjuvants are added to many vaccines to boost the antibody response to the vaccine antigen. Aluminum hydroxide and aluminum sulfate are two metal salts that are frequently used as adjuvants in many different vaccines. One of the first scientists to use aluminum adjuvants in vaccines was Pearl Kendrick, who in the early 1940s demonstrated that aluminum had the power to increase the vaccine's ability to produce antibodies.[45] Kendrick was also instrumental in combining the pertussis whole cell bacteria with tetanus and diphtheria toxoids to form a single vaccine, known today as the DPT. In 1942 Jules Freund and Katherine McDermott developed an oil adjuvant which used tubercule bacilli (tuberculosis germs) to increase the immune response.[46] This product became known as Freund's Adjuvant and has been used widely both in human and animal vaccines.

How Adjuvants Work

Adjuvants work by "trapping" or pooling the vaccine antigen and then dispersing it slowly from the immunization injection site to the lymph nodes and spleen.[47] This process enables vaccine antigens to remain in our body for longer periods of time, thereby stimulating the production of antibodies for longer periods of time. Sometimes vaccine adjuvants are prepared in gels, such as aluminum hydroxide gel. Gels are used for facilitating the dispersal of the vaccine antigen and for providing a medium in which the antigens can be absorbed and protected. Freund's adjuvant is a water-in-oil emulsion consisting of a mineral oil, an antibody stimulator such as tubercule bacilli, and a emulsifying agent such as lanolin or Arlacel A.[48] The vaccine antigens are combined with the adjuvant in a saline solution during vaccine production.

The Adverse Effects of Oil Adjuvants

The main side effects of oil adjuvants have been hypersensitivity reactions, cysts, and adjuvant arthritis. In 1977, Kohashi and associates demonstrated that Freund's adjuvant caused a "delayed" hypersensitivity in rats and caused them to be susceptible to adjuvant arthritis.[49] In 1945 Henle and Henle reported that nodules up to three centimeters in size were found in many individuals immunized with influenza vaccine containing an oil adjuvant. The nodules were present in 40 percent of the vaccinees six months later.[50] In 1956 Pearson noted that oil adjuvants similar to Freund's produced arthritis (inflammation of a joint), synovitis (inflammation of a membrane lining a joint cavity), periostitus (inflammation of a membrane that covers a bone), and tendonitis (inflammation of fibrous cord that attaches muscle to bone) when they were injected within the skin tissue of rats. The rats developed "swelling" in their ankles, paws, tail, and digits fourteen to forty-five days after the oil adjuvant was injected.[51] In 1960, Waksman and colleagues produced an inflammatory condition in test rats, influencing the skin, joints, eyes and mucous membranes, following the inoculation of a tubercule bacilli-in-oil adjuvant.[52]

The adverse reactions to different types of influenza vaccines were noted in an extensive study conducted between 1951 and 1956 and involving 18,000 volunteers.[53] The most visible adverse reaction that occurred from the mineral oil adjuvant in the influenza vaccine was "chronic inflammatory granulomas" that formed at the immunization site.[54] Granulomas are tumors or thick masses of cells that form from granulated tissue.[55] The vaccines were injected into muscle, and the nodules that developed were found "deep in the muscle tissue."[56] What made them a serious consequence of immunization was that the nodules developed into cysts and required heavy drainage, in some cases needing to be surgically removed. The cysts were a long-term effect of influenza immunization, developing within three to twenty-seven months after the immunization.[57] When the cyst fluid was later inspected under a microscope, a large number of mineral oil globules were recovered. Although the cysts were a serious long-term consequence of mineral oil adjuvants, according to the study, only a relatively small number of vacinees, twenty-four in 10,881 (.22 percent) developed them.[58] However, the aqueous influenza vaccine caused systemic reactions (with fever) in 40 percent of the preschool children being tested, and they were receiving only one-fourth to one-half of the adult dosage.[59] In a personal communication from Dr. Jonas Salk to the authors of this study, it was revealed that the emulsifying agent, Arlacel A, used in the oil adjuvants for the year 1951, was found to be "toxic for mice."[60] Although the toxic batch was eliminated, cysts continued to occur. The thousands of people who took part in this vaccine experiment, the majority being children, received this toxic chemical Arlacel A, as did thousands of military recruits at Fort Dix, New Jersey, in 1951.

Although there were serious problems with oil adjuvants such as Freund's Adjuvant, new chemicals, such as aluminum hydroxide, were found to replace old ones. However, twenty-four years after these field studies were performed in 1951, a high-level meeting of the Bureau of Biologics held on November 20, 1975 revealed that the problems inherent in vaccine adjuvants had not been solved. A report of the meeting noted that: "There is little doubt that some of the material containing aluminum as adjuvant appears to be carcinogenic in a strain of Swiss mice. . . . The panel is also investigating the incidence of fibrosarcomas at the usual sites of injections of vaccines."[61]

The use of Freund's adjuvant in millions of doses of vaccines has produced granulomas, cysts, and nodules in a percentage of children and adults receiving them. Although Freund's adjuvant is no longer used in human vaccines, it is still used in animal experiments to produce antibodies. Aluminum hydroxide adjuvants are currently used in vaccines but they are highly suspect of containing carcinogencic (cancerous) material. When heat-killed B pertussis bacteria are combined with aluminum hydroxide (in DPT vaccine) it can produce the potential side effects of complete Freund's adjuvant i.e., granulomas at the injection site.[62]

Both the oil and aluminum adjuvants in vaccines have had a history of producing cysts, nodules, fibromas, fibrosarcomas (malignant tumors), hypersensitivity reactions, and a type of adjuvant arthritis. It appears that the aluminum in vaccines used as adjuvant is not only a contributing factor toward injection-site cysts and granulomas, but may be a contributing factor in cancers and arthritis as well.

FORMALDEHYDE

Formaldehyde is a toxic gaseous compound that is used extensively in both vaccine production and the manufacturing industry. Formaldehyde is utilized in wall and ceiling insulation, its resins are used in the manufacture of wrinkle proof fabrics, and it is a major constituent of embalming fluid.[63] It is also employed in the manufacture of textiles, dyes, inks, and explosives.[64] In medical applications, formaldehyde is used in aqueous solution (i.e., dissolved in water) and used to disinfect excreta and utensils. Formalin, a 37 percent solution of gaseous formaldehyde, which also includes small amounts of methanol, is the chemical of choice used to inactivate the viruses used in the production of polio, yellow fever, influenza, and hepatitis B vaccines. Formalin is also used to detoxify diphtheria and tetanus toxins (in the process changing them to toxoids), a key ingredient of the DPT vaccine. Formalin has had a long history of use in conjunction with vaccines and sera. In 1912 Jules Bordet and Octave Genjou used formaldehyde to "preserve" the first pertussis vaccine.[65] During the 1920s formalin was used extensively in the production of diphtheria toxoid, a product supposedly safer than the deadly toxin antitoxin mixture (TAM) which was in use up to that point.

Adverse Effects of Formaldehyde

Formaldehyde enters the body in three ways: by inhalation, skin contact, and ingestion. The inhalation of formaldehyde causes general irritation to the eyes, nose, and upper respiratory tract.[66] The ingestion of formaldehyde produces a multitude of problems, which may include one or more of the following symptoms: nausea, vomiting, abdominal pain, vertigo, convulsions, coma, severe pain in the mouth and stomach, anuria, and death.[67] The most obvious skin reaction to formaldehyde is an allergic contact dermatitis observed in a percentage of susceptible individuals. After prolonged use, a hardening of the skin occurs.[68] In 1925 Klein reported that the "ingestion" of formaldehyde in the amount of one ounce caused death in three hours.[69] In 1931 Gaal demonstrated that the ingestion of formalin was followed by "inflammation, ulceration and coagulation necrosis" of the gastrointestinal mucosa.[70] Formaldehyde is so toxic that the Environmental Protection Agency has labeled it both a hazardous substance and a hazardous waste.[71]

During the 1970s formaldehyde gas was implicated for causing a wide range of reactions including: headache, nausea, skin rashes, breathing difficulties, and bleeding from the nose.[72] In 1979 the Consumer Product Safety Commission confirmed that small amounts of formaldehyde gas were escaping from foam insulation used in the construction of many residential homes, particularly in the northeast United States. In 1982, as a result, the commission prohibited the use of urea formaldehyde in residential homes and school buildings. In 1977 Hendrick and Lane reported that allergic reactions to formaldehyde occurred in concentrations as low as .8 parts per million.[73] The most damaging evidence of formaldehyde poisoning has come in recent years from the Chemical Industries Institute and was confirmed by scientists at New York University. Their investigations revealed that inhaled formaldehyde gas produced squanomous cell carcinomas (cancers) in the nasal cavaties of rats.[74]

Doubtful Abilities of Formalin

There are numerous problems associated with using formalin in vaccine production. First, there is the poisoning effect. Second, there is formalin's inability to adequately disinfect, i.e., render the viral and bacterial antigens in vaccines safe for human use. This last point was a hot topic of debate in the years preceding and following the use of the Salk polio vaccine in April 1955. M.V. Veldee, M.D., then chairman of the biology department at Stanford Research Institute, expressed grave doubts that polio vaccine could ever uniformly be made safe for human use, using formalin as the inactivating agent. In a commentary published in the *New England Journal of Medicine* in September 1955, Dr. Veldee gave his reasons. During the production of polio vaccine, he said, vaccine particles become trapped within a protein "gelantinous" material, an effect known as "clumping."[75] The action of formalin on this material tends to solidify it—thus protecting it from the inactivating wash of the disinfectant.[76] Once the polio vaccine antigens are injected inside the human body this "coating" is ingested by enzymes allowing the virus particles to escape.[77] These living vaccine viral antigens have the ability to cause or activate polio in the child, to a lesser or greater degree, depending on how virulent the viral antigens are, the amount of virus received, and how well the child's immune system can cope with the insult. In any event, this is a dangerous situation, and none of it is supposed to happen.

Another difficult problem associated with formalin in vaccine production is determining the right amount to use. If not enough formalin is used, virulent virus particles in the vaccine culture broth will remain alive, untouched by the neutralizing wash of formalin. If too much formalin is used it will jeopardize the potency of the vaccine—in some cases completely inactivating the viral antigen.

The Cutter Incident

The suspicions of Dr. Veldee concerning the doubtful abilities of formalin to inactivate polio virus effectively proved to be true. Just two to three weeks after the first Salk polio vaccine was injected into millions of American children in April 1955, clusterings of paralytic polio cases began to be reported in different parts of the United States, not only in children having just received the vaccine but also in their family and community contacts. A number of researchers (Timm, Haas, Wessler) investigated the polio disaster and discovered that formalin was uniformly ineffective as a disinfectant in the presence of protein.[78] In 1955 Scheele reported that formalin failed to inactivate some batches of virulent polio vaccine even when the procedure was repeated two or three times.[79]

The results of the first Salk polio vaccine campaign, in which five million children were immunized, were tabulated in 1963 by Nathanson and Langmuir. According to their investigation, the vaccine caused 260 cases of polio of which 192 (74 percent) were paralytic.[80] A further breakdown of cases revealed that 94 cases occurred in vaccinated people, of which 59 (63 percent) were paralytic; 126 cases occurred in family contacts of which 101 were paralytic (80 percent) and 40 cases occurred in community contacts, of which 32 (80 percent) were paralytic.[81] Ten deaths occurred. As a result, sixty lawsuits were brought against Cutter Laboratories, of which fifty-four had been settled by April 1962 for an aggregate amount in excess of three million dollars.[82]

The inability of formaldehyde to uniformly inactivate large batches of seed virus, thus exposing people unexpectedly to vaccines that are completely unfit for use in humans, may be the ultimate irony. Here we have a chemical, formaldehyde, designated by the EPA as a hazardous substance and hazardous waste, being used by scientists to make a vaccine safe. Could there be a more ridiculous, warped idea? Even more significant is the almost unbelievable notion of using a substance as deadly as formaldehyde, in any amount, as part of a preventive medicine. What sane person would consider using a hazardous waste, carcinogenic in rats, used in the manufacture of inks, dyes, explosives, wrinkle-proof fabrics, home insulation, and as a major constitutent of embalming fluid, and inject it into the delicate body of an infant? What could formaldehyde, aluminum, phenol, mercury, or any number of other deadly chemical substances used in vaccines possibly have to do with preventing disease in children? The fact that they are needed at all in the vaccine formula argues that the product is toxic, unstable, and unreliable with or without their presence.

The Inherent Toxicity of Vaccine Preservatives

While many of the toxic substances found in vaccines, such as aluminum, formalin, thimerosal, and mineral oil adjuvants are clearly dangerous for humans to ingest, and have been proven so by numerous scientific studies, it is almost impossible to find one article in any medical journal that incriminates vaccines for being inherently toxic drugs. In 1971 Marcus Mason, John Baker, and C.C. Cate performed extensive studies with seven compounds commonly used as preservatives or extracting agents in the preparation of vaccines.[83] The chemicals were: merthiolate (thimerosal), benzethonium chloride, methyl paraben, phenol red, pyridine, ethylene glycol, and ethylene chlorohydrin. The goal of the study was to determine the acute lethal dose of each compound (LD 50), the maximum tolerated dose, and the carcinogenicity of the compounds.

During the experiments, test rats were divided into groups, with each group receiving two weekly injections (.25 ml. per injection) of a specific chemical for a full year. The animals were then observed for another year. Three types of control groups were used in the study: a vehicle control group which received .25 ml. injections of saline, a negative control which received no drug treatment, and a positive control group which received injections of nickel sulfide.

Thimerosal, a common preservative used in many vaccines, caused severe lesions in the rats' lungs affecting their "defense apparatus" and produced a high incidence of bronchopneumonia.[84] After twelve months of drug treatment and six months of observation, thimerosal produced the highest mortality among the seven chemicals tested, 9 percent. The authors suggest that the damage caused by thimerosal may be cumulative. Although all the chemicals produced deaths in the animals, it must be recognized that the negative control group, which received no drug treatment, had a death rate of 5.8 percent.

In evaluating the carcinogenic potential of the chemicals, benzethonium chloride produced indurations or sarcomas at the injection site in 13 percent of the test animals.[85] Thimerosal produced the second highest number of fibromas and produced many injection-site indurations.[86] The other compounds produced tumors at the rate of 1 to 2 percent. The majority of the tumors were fibrosarcomas, which are malignant tumors likely to have a fatal outcome. Overall, mammary fibroadenomas occurred at the rate of 2 to 5 percent and uterine polyps occurred in 4 to 11 percent of the test rats (and in 10 percent of the controls).[87]

All seven chemicals produced tumors not only at the injection site, but also in other parts of the body. There were eighteen pituitary tumors (adenomas), eight adrenal tumors, and seventeen blood tumors (leukemias), for an additional forty-three tumors seen in 1,620 rats.[88] In the positive control group, nickel sulfide produced the greatest number of tumors. Rats that received no drug treatment or ones who received injections of saline also produced some tumors, but in smaller numbers than those receiving the vaccine preservatives.

It was the opinion of the authors that the high rate of tumors following the injection of benzethonium chloride was a significant finding and was related to the amount of the test dose. They said, "The correlation is great between a very high rate of initial irritation, subsequent granulomas, and the gradual development of massive tumors."[89]

The Mason, Baker and Cate study, one of the few studies that tested certain preservatives and extracting agents used in the preparation of vaccines, found that all seven compounds produced tumors in test rats. Thimerosal and bezethonium chloride produced sarcomas and injection site indurations. Indurations (or hard nodules that appear at the injection site) are an aftereffect of influenza, DPT, and other vaccines.

Can there be any doubt that at least three chemicals used in vaccines: thimerosal, bezethonium chloride, and aluminum are probable causes of induration, fibromas, fibrasarcomas, granulomas, and injection site tumors? If these chemicals have already produced all manner of tumors in test animals, and vaccines are already known causes of indurations and injection site granulomas, then it is hard to escape the conclusion that vaccines, or some of the material contained in them, may be a prime cause of cancer and leukemia.

The toxicity of aluminum, formaldehyde, and thimerosal is well established among toxicologists, yet few parallels have been drawn to the damaging effect these chemicals might have on children. Even more alarming is the cumulative effect they might have on a baby over time. Therefore, it is reasonable to think that the amount of chemicals used in vaccines may induce serious toxic allergic/hypersensitivity reactions in infants, especially when they are receiving ten or more vaccine injections before they are barely eighteen months old; and in light of their small size, low body weight, and relatively immature and developing immune system.

The use of hazardous chemicals in vaccine production helps to further define the true nature of a vaccine. Are vaccines really a life-saving, disease-preventing miracle of science? Or are they something entirely more sinister, masquerading as a great medical discovery?

It may well be that vaccines are the starting ground for other current diseases of unknown origins, for which medical science cannot find either cause or cure.

CHAPTER 7

The Provocation Effect of Vaccines and Other Drugs

*I*n addition to the carcinogenic potential of many vaccine chemicals is the mechanism by which these chemicals may be inciting infections and disease. Medical literature has, in abundance, examples of the effects of certain drugs or irritating substances in causing allergic reactions, anaphylactic shock, convulsions, or provoking the onset of certain disease conditions. In 1954 a study published in the *Lancet* briefly reviewed a half-century of research outlining the diverse factors that provoke or increase the severity of polio in its victims, or localize it to a certain section in the nervous system. Some of those factors included: vaccination, trauma, tonsillectomies, pertussis vaccines, and the injection of numerous substances such as cortisone, bismuth, guanine, and penicillin.[1]

During the early days of polio research at the turn of the twentieth century, there was clinical evidence that the polio virus traveled through the body via the circulatory system. This provided a basis for researchers Trueta and Hodes to suggest that perhaps all the diverse factors that influence the severity and localization of polio might have an element in common: namely that they somehow modify the pattern of blood vessels in the nervous system thereby increasing the permeability of the blood-brain barrier, thus giving polio virus easier access to the nervous system and brain. In order to demonstrate their hypothesis, the authors concentrated on the effects of two irritating substances: formalin-saline and croton oil.

In one experiment a 10 percent solution of formalin-saline (.05 ml) was injected into the right hind leg of a mouse. Within one hour, the mouse's leg became paralyzed and four days later, the mouse was dead.[2] The same results occurred when a 1 percent solution of formalin-saline in the amount of .05 ml was injected. The authors showed convincing evidence, enhanced by photographs, that the blood vessels in the spinal cord tree became "engorged" specifically on the right side, corresponding to the right leg of the mouse.[3] Similar results were obtained with rabbits when a .5 ml injection of 1 in 50 croton oil was inoculated into their thighs. It was clear from photographs that sections of the spinal cord most affected were areas supplying nerves to the "injected limb."[4]

Trueta and Hodes demonstrated that at least two irritating substances might increase the permeability of the blood-brain barrier affecting the severity and localization of the disease in question, polio. They give credit to researchers such as Amoss, Flexner, Speransky, Millet, and LeFevre de Arric, who preceded them in this line of work and whose own work revealed that certain diverse factors such as trauma, intraspinal injections, and irritating substances injected under the skin or into the muscle increase the permeability of the blood-brain barrier, thereby provoking or increasing the severity of disease caused by pathogens.[5] When these irritating substances were combined with disease pathogens and injected into test animals, their ability to provoke or increase the severity of disease was undeniable—especially in comparison to control animals not receiving the substances. Trueta and Hodes reported that:

"When the diverse influences were combined with the injection of the casual agents of poliomyelitis, herpes, rabies, and tetanus, death or serious disease resulted, whereas control animals not so treated, either presented significantly reduced symptoms or were entirely free from the clinical disease."[6]

Vaccines and Other Drugs
Provoke Paralytic Polio

In 1953 Rosen and Thooris provided powerful evidence that irritating substances significantly increase the chances of paralysis from polio.   They reported that during a polio epidemic in French Oceania, children under the age of fifteen, who were receiving weekly injections of mercury, arsenic, and bismuth to combat treponematosis, (an infestation of the same family of spirochetes that cause syphilis and yaws) experienced paralytic polio at ten times the rate of children not receiving the treatments.[7]

Other evidence reveals that heavy metals, vaccines, or formalin may provoke paralytic polio or other acute disease processes.   During the 1940s and 1950s children who were recently vaccinated with pertussis vaccines suffered a substantially increased incidence of paralytic polio.   During a polio outbreak in Minnesota in 1946, of eighty-five confirmed cases of paralytic polio, thirty-three cases had been recently inoculated with pertussis vaccine.[8]   In these cases, paralytic polio followed within five to nineteen days after inoculation and the injected limb was paralyzed in 58 percent of the cases.[9]   Benjamin and Gore, who did extensive studies on the relationship between pertussis vaccines and paralytic polio, said, for the year 1949, the risk of contracting paralytic polio for infants aged nine to twenty-four months was four times higher if they had received an injection of diphtheria-pertussis vaccine within the last six weeks, as compared to an uninoculated control group of infants.[10]   In 1954 the Medical Research Council of Great Britain conducted a study that demonstrated conclusively that pertussis vaccines, especially the aluminum-precipitated diphtheria pertussis vaccine, can "predispose" a child to paralytic polio disease.[11]   In 1957, René Dubos, the renowned microbiologist, proved experimentally that when pertussis vaccines or killed mycobacteria were injected into animals who had been infected months earlier with small doses of bacteria, the numbers of bacteria multiplied explosively in the animals, and many died.   The pertussis vaccine and the mycobacteria were able to accelerate latent infections into acute infections.[12]   Bodian believed that the vaccines cause a change in the blood vessels of the spinal cord, allowing the vaccine virus to penetrate more easily.[13]   Graham Wilson, M.D., author of *The Hazards of*

Immunization, commented that this provocation disease or provocation effect brought on by many vaccines usually occurs when the patient, especially during polio, is in the incubation stage of the disease or has some latent infection which the vaccine or medication reactivates, perhaps by lowering the tissue resistance of the host.[14] Ralph Scobey, M.D., has even postulated that polio is not an infectious disease and is caused by a number of factors all of which produce a direct poisoning effect.[15]

In any event, it has been shown that certain drugs, chemicals, and irritating substances injected under the skin, such as formalin, croton oil, mercury, bismuth, penicillin, guanine, cortisone, pertussis vaccines, have caused an increase of paralysis and death both experimentally in animals and in humans with polio. Since medical science has failed to reach any singular conclusion as to why so many people in every country of the world employing immunization have suffered adverse vaccine reactions, clearly it is time that a direct connection be made between these reactions and vaccine preservatives, germicides, cationic surficants, antibiotics, aluminum-containing adjuvants and other irritating substances.

CHAPTER 8

The Decline of Childhood Diseases Before Vaccination

O ne of the distinctions vaccination has claimed for itself is that it is largely responsible for reducing the incidence and mortality of the major childhood diseases of this century. This sweeping claim, fostered by many in the medical profession and believed by unsuspecting millions, has been used ad infinitum by the profession to justify the success of vaccine programs and to further their continued use. After reading other writers who presented factual evidence that many childhood diseases decreased in morbidity and mortality long before the advent of mass immunizations, I decided to investigate the matter.

From 1911 to 1935, the four leading causes of death among those aged one to fourteen, covered by Metropolitan Life Insurance Company policies, were (1) diphtheria, (2) measles, (3) scarlet fever, (4) and whooping cough.[1] The standardized death rate among children ages one to fourteen from the leading childhood diseases declined from 145 per 100,000 living in 1911, to 28 per 100,000 in 1935, a decrease of 81 percent.[2] By 1945, the annual death rate from the four leading communicable diseases of childhood had declined to 7 per 100,000.[3] Thus, the combined death rate of diphtheria, measles, scarlet fever, and whooping cough declined 95 percent among children ages one to fourteen from 1911 to 1945, before the mass immunization programs started in the United States.

MEASLES

Measles ranks second as a cause of death among the four leading childhood diseases prevalent between 1911 and 1935. The death rate for measles decreased from 27 per 100,000 in 1911, to 6 per 100,000 in 1935, a decline in mortality of 77 percent.[4]

Mortality figures from twenty-two American cities revealed that measles deaths decreased steadily from 1887 to 1935, with most of the decrease occurring before 1920.[5] The measles vaccine was introduced in 1963, so any assertion that measles vaccination had a hand in the decrease in mortality is completely unfounded. If the vaccine could not have been responsible, why did measles deaths decline so significantly? Louis Dublin and Alfred Lotka, statisticians and authors of the comprehensive studies done at Metropolitan Life Insurance Company in 1937, remark that the decline in measles mortality was due to "better nutrition, improved physical conditions, better hygienic surroundings, and more adequate medical and nursing care during illness and convalescence."[6] They continue, " The use of convalescent serum is both too recent and too limited to explain any substantial part of the downward trend."[7] George Bigelow, M.D., chairman of the White House Committee on Communicable Disease Control in 1931, commented that during the 1920s while the general mortality from measles was only 5 to 10 deaths per 100,000, the case-fatality rates (or the proportion of cases of a specified disease which are fatal within a specified time), perhaps reached 35 percent in infant asylums due to "the prevalence of rickets and other forms of malnutrition, the overcrowding, and inadequate nursing and hygienic care."[8] Furthermore, he notes that "higher fatality rates among Negroes and Indians are more likely due to living conditions, and inadequate medical and nursing care, than to inherent hypersusceptibility."[9] These observations were significant, not only for the time period in which they were made, but also for the present; and they will be helpful later on when we evaluate the increased incidence of measles cases in the United States since 1983.

SCARLET FEVER

Scarlet fever had the third highest death rate among the communicable diseases of childhood. A survey of twenty-one American cities revealed that during the period 1885 to 1933, the crude death rate from scarlet fever dropped sharply from 40 per 100,000 to 12 per 100,000 in just the four-year period between 1892 and 1896.[10] Overall, the death rate from scarlet fever declined steadily from 1892 to 1935. Among Metropolitan policyholders ages one to fourteen, the death rate from scarlet fever decreased from 27 per 100,000 in 1911, to 7 per 100,000 in 1935, a decrease of 73 percent.[11] According to Dublin, convalescent serums, which were available in the 1920s and 1930s to "temper" the severity of scarlet fever, at best, only provided temporary immunity. Because the serums were not used on a grand scale, there is no evidence that they had any significant effect on the decrease in mortality from scarlet fever.[12]

WHOOPING COUGH (PERTUSSIS)

Although physicians have found no cure for whooping cough, its incidence and mortality have declined from the mid-nineteenth century to the mid-twentieth century. During the period 1885 to 1933, the crude death rate for whooping cough, decreased (in an up-and-down pattern) from 21 deaths per 100,000 in 1886, to 6 deaths per 100,000 in 1904.[13] After 1904, a similar pattern of decline continued until about 1920, after which the decrease became more uniform, continuing to the year 1933.[14] Among Metropolitan policyholders ages one to fourteen, the death rate from whooping cough declined from 19 per 100,000 in 1911, to 5 per 100,000 in 1935, a decrease in mortality of 73 percent.[15]

Since 1935 the death rate for whooping cough has continued to decline, not only in the United States, but in the countries of Western Europe as well. In Sweden there were 800 whooping cough deaths per year between 1911 and 1915, yet only 10 deaths from 1951 to 1955.[16] Mass immunization programs for whooping cough did not begin in Sweden until the mid-1950s, and so the continued decrease in mortality to very low levels occurred before vaccinations commenced. In Hamburg, Germany the picture is similar. There were 986 deaths from among 7,716 cases of whooping cough between 1901 and 1905. However, there were only 33 deaths among 11,123 cases between 1951 and 1955.[17] No doubt the decrease in mortality from whooping cough before mass immunizations was due to better housing, better nutrition, less crowding in the home, and other hygienic, nursing, or public health improvements. Antibiotics also helped reduce the mortality from whooping cough by controlling "secondary infections" such as bronchitis and pneumonia, thus giving babies a higher chance of surviving the illness.[18]

DIPHTHERIA

The death rate for diphtheria was the highest among the four leading communicable diseases of childhood between 1911 and 1935. Despite this, the mortality from diphtheria decreased from 72 deaths per 100,000 in 1911, to 9 deaths per 100,000 in 1935, a decrease of 88 percent.[19] Dublin and Lotka credit diphtheria antitoxin as a major reason for the decrease in mortality. In New York City, where diphtheria was prevalent and deaths as numerous as anywhere in the United States, antitoxin was used to immunize school children on a limited scale beginning in 1920.[20] By 1934, an estimated 45 percent of preschool children attending New York City schools had been immunized against diphtheria.[21] While the number of diphtheria cases (all ages) declined in the boroughs of Manhattan and the Bronx from 3,854 in 1929 to 686 in 1934, and deaths declined from 190 to 32, the case-fatality rate remained unchanged, hovering around 5 percent.[22] While the morbidity and mortality of diphtheria certainly declined in New York City during the diphtheria antitoxin campaign, the mortality from diphtheria had been declining since 1881.[23] Between 1881 and 1898 deaths from diphtheria in children less than ten years old decreased dramatically in New York City from 1,200 per 100,000 to 210 per 100,000.[24] After 1898, deaths from diphtheria continued to decline steadily up to 1935 and beyond.

Because the decline in deaths from diphtheria began many years before antitoxin was first used in 1895, used on a limited scale in the years before and after 1920, and on a wide scale in the late 1930s and early 1940s, to say that antitoxin or toxoid was responsible for the decline is clearly missing the point. Although the number of cases dropped more rapidly perhaps after vaccinations began, diphtheria had been declining for many years before that time.   My view is that diphtheria antitoxin or toxoid did little to alter the course of diphtheria in a positive way.

Conversely, some other pertinent facts about diphtheria antitoxin suggest that it may have actually increased deaths. Antitoxin is given to patients to destroy the toxin that circulates in the blood after someone becomes infected with diphtheria. However, the antitoxin does not destroy toxin that has "already been bound to tissue," producing damage.[25] How many untold numbers of people receiving antiserum were in this position? Additionally, many cases of diphtheria and subsequent deaths followed the immediate use of diphtheria toxin-antitoxin mixture (TAM).   In 1919, in Dallas, Texas, an unknown number of children, estimated as at least 84, had severe reactions to diphtheria toxin-antitoxin mixture following the administration of the vaccine.[26] In 1948, in Kyoto, Japan, more than 600 infants became severely ill, resulting in 68 deaths, after the infants were injected with alum-precipitated diphtheria toxoid.[27]

When one considers that the incidence and mortality from diphtheria declined before antitoxin was used, and, a lesser known fact, that serious cases of diphtheric poisoning occurred from the vaccine, it seems more than likely that the large decline in mortality from diphtheria between 1911 and 1935 was due to other health factors such as: less crowding in the home, better nutrition, and other public health measures, which insured that diphtheria declined by itself.

Thus it is evident that all of the four leading causes of death in children declined in incidence and mortality long before vaccines were introduced on a mass scale. The influence of factors such as decreased overcrowding in homes and improved nutrition and hygiene cannot be ignored.

CHAPTER 9

Whooping Cough in Vaccinated and Unvaccinated Children

During the 1920s and 1930s, whooping cough (pertussis) was prevalent in the United States, especially among children under five. During this time a number of well-managed studies were undertaken by the Public Health Service to determine the incidence and mortality of whooping cough in different parts of the United States. In addition, other controlled field trials provided data on the effectiveness of the pertussis vaccine. These studies provide a fairly accurate assessment of whooping cough as it occurred in small villages, towns, and large cities in the United States during various times between 1922 and 1936, before the advent of pertussis vaccine.

RURAL TOWNS AND CITIES 1922-1932

The first surveys that evaluated the incidence and mortality of whooping cough took place in Hagerstown, Maryland, and upstate New York.[1] A second study, known as the "Costs of Medical Care," surveyed the incidence of whooping cough among large numbers of people in eighteen states.[2] The number of cases uncovered by the two studies was moderately high although not unusual for that time period: 747 cases among 16,981 people, and 1,588 cases among 42,971 people.[3] However, what is striking is the low number of deaths. Of the 1,588 cases of pertussis in the second study, only three died. In 1933 whooping cough accounted for 4,463 deaths among 1,342,106 deaths from all causes in the registration area of the continental United States.[4] During the 1930s, perhaps 50 percent of whooping cough deaths were in children less than one year old, and as many as 95 percent of deaths were in children less than five years old.[5] It is easy to see why extra protection was sought for this age group of infants and children. If an infant escaped death, secondary complications of whooping cough, including bronchitis, pneumonia, middle ear infections, and blindness were not uncommon. The Committee on Communicable Disease Control, made up of leading physicians on child health and organized in response to the White House Conference on Child Health and Protection under President Herbert Hoover in 1930, made some insightful statements about the state of whooping cough in the late 1920s, and also about pertussis vaccine, which had been used on a limited scale up to that point. Its first observation was that whooping cough was "especially fatal in rachitic (rickets-suffering) and undernourished children living under unhygienic conditions."[6] Secondly, "the immunizing value of whooping cough vaccine is doubtful both as to degree and duration."[7] These statements, made at a time when whooping cough posed a significant threat to vulnerable children, will be helpful a little later on when we look at the results of other studies that evaluated the protective value of pertussis vaccines both in that era and in later years.

CLEVELAND, OHIO 1934-1936

During the 1930s, field trials with pertussis vaccines were carried out in different cities, notably Cleveland, Ohio; Binghamton, New York; and Grand Rapids, Michigan. The study performed in Cleveland between 1934 and 1936 tested the effectiveness of pertussis vaccine on a group of 483 infants, ranging in age from 6 to 15 months.[8] A group of 496 non-vaccinated infants was used as the control. The study was carefully monitored by physicians and nurses for more than two years. The most surprising test result was that whooping cough attacked both groups of children equally; there were 71 cases among 496 unvaccinated infants, and 61 cases among 483 vaccinated infants.[9] There was only one death occurring in an unvaccinated infant among 132 cases of whooping cough.[10]

One of the main justifications for using a vaccine is that it must protect its recipients from the disease in question. A second criterion is that the vaccine must achieve better results than the natural disease unhindered. In this case, the pertussis vaccine failed to give any better results than those experienced by the unvaccinated children; there was no appreciable difference in either the attack rates or the mortality from pertussis in vaccinated and unvaccinated children.

BINGHAMTON, NEW YORK 1939-1940

The protective capabilities of pertussis vaccines were evaluated in a study done in Binghamton, New York from 1939 to 1940.[11] When both vaccinated and unvaccinated children were exposed to whooping cough in their environment, some from within their households and others from contacts outside the home, both groups developed pertussis to varying degrees. Among forty-four vaccinated children exposed to pertussis, 32 percent developed the clinical disease.[12] Among the forty-six unvaccinated children, 72 percent developed pertussis.[13]

The next test evaluation was the secondary attack rate—or the number of children or adults who contracted pertussis and who also lived in the same households as their source contact (who were known or suspected to have pertussis). Under these circumstances, among vaccinated children, eighteen secondary cases resulted from fifty-three definite or suspected source cases. Among the unvaccinated, forty-six secondary household attacks occurred from fifty-eight known or suspected source cases. Overall, the secondary attack rate in vaccinated children was 34 percent and the secondary attack rate in unvaccinated children was 79 percent.[14]

This study demonstrates that the number of pertussis cases occurring in unvaccinated children was more than two times the number occurring in vaccinated children. If taken on face value, however, these figures are misleading. I say that with confidence because as the Cleveland study has shown, whooping cough attacked vaccinated and unvaccinated children equally. In the Binghamton study, more unvaccinated children got the disease. The numbers sometimes favor the vaccinated and other times the unvaccinated. The question one should ask is: What is the true protective value of the pertussis vaccine? How effective is the vaccine when 32 percent of fully vaccinated children known to have been exposed to whooping cough developed the clinical disease and 34 percent of household contacts or secondary attack rates occurred in fully vaccinated infants and children. Where is the protection for these children? How well is pertussis vaccine working, if at all? I believe this is why Dr. Bigelow and leading physicians of the 1920s and 1930s remarked that pertussis vaccine was "doubtful as to degree and duration."

PERTUSSIS VACCINE IN GREAT BRITAIN 1942-1978

Some of the first trials in Europe with pertussis vaccines were carried out in England between 1942 and 1944 by the Medical Research Council. It tested the protective powers of pertussis vaccine on nursery school children in Oxford, Berkshire, and Buckinghamshire, England (see table 9-1). As the table shows, whooping cough attacked both vaccinated and unvaccinated children equally. The authors concluded that there was "no significant difference in the incidence and severity of [whooping cough] between the vaccinated and unvaccinated groups. . . . and that no satisfactory evidence was obtained that the vaccine was of any value in modifying the course of the disease."[15] This statement not only confirms the results of the Cleveland study and the Costs of Medical Care Survey in the United States, but also adds a valuable piece of information that has been generally overlooked by health departments; i.e., that vaccines (in this case pertussis vaccine) fail to modify the course of a disease.

During the 1960s and 1970s, two leading European physicians, Dr. Justus Strom of the Hospital of Infectious Diseases in Stockholm, Sweden, and Dr. Gordon Stewart, professor of community medicine at the University of Glasgow, Scotland, began to question the use of mass pertussis vaccine programs in their respective countries, especially when the natural course of pertussis had become milder in both countries, and the death

Table 9-1

INCIDENCE OF WHOOPING-COUGH, REGARDLESS OF HISTORY OF EXPOSURE, AMONG ALL CHILDREN IN THE INVESTIGATION

	OXFORD CITY		RESIDENTIAL NURSERIES	
	Inoculated Children	Control Children	Inoculated Children	Control Children
Number of children observed	327	305	33	30
Number of cases of definite whooping cough	41	43	18	19
Number of cases of doubtful whooping cough	10	6	5	3
Proportion of children with definite whooping cough	12.5%	14.1%	54.6%	63.3%

Source: A.M. McFarlan, E. Topley, and M. Fisher, "Trial of Whooping-Cough Vaccine in City and Residential Nursery Groups," *British Medical Journal* 1 (August 18, 1945): 207-208.

rate from pertussis was very small. In addition, the neurological complications from the vaccine seemed to be more widespread than anyone imagined. These complications were not being taken seriously enough by the medical profession to serve as a prime deterrent for administering pertussis vaccines further to all children on a mass scale. In 1977, Dr. Stewart reported that pertussis disease declined in incidence and mortality in Glasgow, during "epidemic years" from 1900 to 1957.[16] After 1957, the year mass vaccination for pertussis began in England and Scotland, the decline continued. Stewart also noted, citing the official records of the registrar-general, that the same decline in pertussis morbidity and mortality occurred in England and Wales from 1929 to 1957, in both cases, decades before the use of pertussis vaccines on a mass scale. Other revelations made by Dr. Stewart concerning pertussis vaccines in his native Scotland were both revealing and incriminating for the vaccine.

In a study comparing different aspects of pertussis in vaccinated and unvaccinated children, in family, school, and hospital settings during 1974 and 1975, Stewart revealed that there was no difference between the duration of illness, the severity of illness, the general incidence of whooping cough, or the number of primary or secondary cases of whooping cough in vaccinated or unvaccinated children.[17] In the family study, cases of whooping cough occurring in fully vaccinated older people accounted for 68 percent of the cases.[18] Statistics drawn from absentee records of ten primary schools revealed that 61 percent of whooping cough cases occurred in children who had received a full course of DPT vaccine.[19] Additionally, in secondary cases of pertussis, 70 percent of the "introducers" were fully vaccinated, as were 48 percent of their contacts.[20] Again, this important statistic deflates the theory that vaccinated infants provide immunity to older children who in turn become "less infectious" to other infants.

By 1967, the efficacy of the DPT vaccine or the triple vaccine, as it is called in England and Wales, had reached an all-time low of 20 percent.[21] This means the vaccine protected from clinical disease only one-fifth of the children receiving it. The key words here are "clinical disease" or the normal observable symptoms of disease, for the efficacy of a vaccine is measured in terms of how well it prevents clinical disease, not how well it prevents infection.[22] This distinction is an important one, especially since pertussis has become milder in recent decades and may be underreported as a result. As recently as 1991, in a study investigating an outbreak of pertussis in Pembrokeshire, England, one more mystery about vaccine effectiveness was finally solved. "Notified cases [those reported by medical doctors] were significantly less likely to have been vaccinated than other cases with similar symptoms. Therefore, vaccine efficacy estimates based upon notified cases are likely to be biased."[23] This means that most cases of pertussis, when reported by physicians, are in children who are unvaccinated. The author learned upon investigation that there were similar cases in vaccinated children not being reported. Because vaccine efficacy is measured as protection from clinical disease in vaccinated children as compared to unvaccinated children, this statistical glitch could very easily give a vaccine efficacy rate for pertussis or any other vaccine that is higher than the efficacy really is. Secondly, because efficacy counts only clinical cases (some vaccinated, some not), and thousands more children have milder cases, there is great room for dishonest reporting to the public that vaccines have a high success rate, when the evidence shows that they have a moderate to poor success rate.

The mark of vaccine effectiveness is not only how well it protects children from disease, but also how well mass immunization programs reduce the transmission of disease in a population. In England and Wales, epidemics of whooping cough have continued to occur like clockwork every three or four years from before the pertussis vaccine was introduced into Great Britain throughout the years of maximum vaccinations.[24] By 1974, pertussis vaccination levels in England and Wales had dropped dramatically from about 75 to 85 percent of children during the 1960s, to about 30 percent, and remained at that level through 1978 and thereafter.[25] This reduction in the number of vaccinated children introduced a large influx of susceptible children (unvaccinated) into the childhood population pool and according to "classical" theory should have led to a shortened time interval between the year low vaccination rates began in 1974, and the next epidemic of whooping cough. However, paradoxically, it did not. The next whooping cough epidemic occurred in England in 1978, four years after the last one.[26]

There is much to say about this event and certainly room for a variety of interpretations. My view is that pertussis epidemics, like measles epidemics, (which have also occurred with remarkable regularity from before measles vaccines were introduced through times of high vaccine intake), are cyclical diseases and are beyond the manipulation of scientists to alter their course with mass vaccination programs. Therefore, in 1978, all the allegedly susceptible unvaccinated children in England, whose numbers had increased considerably during the previous four years, did not cause an epidemic of whooping cough to occur any sooner; children are only as vulnerable to whooping cough as their individual health and environment allow. Regardless of other factors, they all have natural immunity to protect them, whether they are vaccinated or not.

During the 1970s, as news of serious neurological complications following the use of DPT vaccine became more widespread in Western Europe, far fewer parents vaccinated their children against diphtheria, pertussis, and tetanus. A third aspect of this changing scenario was that natural whooping cough disease became milder in England, Wales, Scotland, Sweden, and West Germany. In Sweden, there were 19,000 reported cases of pertussis between 1977 and 1979, yet not a single child died as a result.[27] Whooping cough was no longer a threatening disease in Sweden, even for infants, who are the most vulnerable to it. John Taranger of the Vastra Frolunda Hospital in Sweden remarked in 1982 that no child has died from pertussis in Sweden since 1970.[28] At the same time in Glasgow, Scotland, a city of about a million people, there have been no deaths from pertussis since 1971.[29] Because whooping cough has become milder in some countries of Europe, since about 1970, and because of the ineffectiveness of the triple vaccine, DPT vaccination was halted in West Germany in 1976 and in Sweden in 1979.[30,31]

One of the major pitfalls of pertussis vaccines has been their inability to prevent the observable, clinical form of whooping cough with much consistency. Vaccine efficacy levels for pertussis vaccines have fluctuated wildly over the years (20 to 75 percent in England, 63 to 94 percent in the United States), such that, on any given day, it does not protect children very well from whooping cough. In addition, five DPT shots are required between the ages of two months and four years to gain and maintain immunity. This indicates how fleeting vaccine immunity really is. Alarmingly, some 45 to 95 percent of all people who receive the full course of DPT vaccinations are still susceptible to whooping cough—for up to twelve years afterwards.[32] Second attacks following natural whooping cough have been described as rare.[33]

It is my opinion that thousands of infants and children develop mild or subclinical infections to pertussis bacteria each year; some are unvaccinated children who "catch" the disease naturally through exposure, and the remainder are vaccinated children who develop the disease either directly from DPT inoculation or from exposure in the environment. This second way occurs because the DPT vaccine simply fails to protect against whooping cough in a good many cases. Most do not see doctors for the disease specifically, and perhaps only a fraction are recognized having "true" cases of whooping cough confirmed by blood test and culture. The remainder of cases are probably diagnosed as some kind of respiratory infection. If the children were immunized for DPT and later develop the symptomatology of pertussis, they will not likely be diagnosed as having whooping cough, but rather some other similar respiratory infection. Misdiagnosis will occur, especially if they do not exhibit the characteristic "whoop," but is more likely because many doctors are still slow to diagnose a disease in a child vaccinated against it. Whooping cough tends to be milder in a vaccinated child and indeed it may not be recognizable as such. Perhaps, the DPT vaccine containing the pertussis whole cell bacteria, tetanus and diphtheria toxoids and other toxic preservatives and germicides, alters the child's natural immune response, producing a mild, subclinical, atypical, or abortive new infection in its place.

What all this means to me is that the DPT vaccine is grossly ineffective. Judging from the vaccine's historical track record, people might feel justified in flipping a coin in deciding whether to vaccinate their child. And yet we're still basing that decision on vaccine efficacy—a numbers game fraught with inaccuracies. If the decision to vaccinate a child really is a numbers game, advantages versus risks, then the most important numbers have yet to be entered into the equation—the known risk of vaccine reactions.

CHAPTER 10

The Adverse Reactions to Vaccines

*E*ver since childhood vaccines came into use, there have been children in whom the vaccine didn't "take" properly. In some cases, this meant that the vaccine failed to protect the child against the disease he or she was vaccinated against. During the 1970s and 1980s, many children who received the measles vaccine at the recommended age contracted measles later on—as school-age children, adolescents, or adults.[1]

In other cases, the vaccine itself gave children the disease. This type of disaster occurred in 1955 after the mass inoculation of five million school children with Salk inactivated polio vaccine. As a result, there were 260 reported cases of polio occurring within three to twenty-five days after the injection. The reason for the catastrophe was that certain batches of polio vaccine, not being completely inactivated during production, became destructive to nerve tissue.[2]

In a third type of vaccination failure, some component of the vaccine caused an allergic reaction or a systemic poisoning effect, producing a wide range of symptom/reactions, which ran the gamut from sore arms to collapse and death.

The types of vaccine reactions suffered in children are so numerous and varied that they require different classifications. In general, there are three categories of vaccine reactions: local, systemic, and neurological.

Local Reaction

A local reaction affects the area immediately around the inoculation site, which is usually on the arm or leg, but may also be the buttocks. These reactions are primarily skin reactions, which may produce pain, redness, soreness, swelling, and tenderness. While most of the uncomfortable effects of the vaccine subside within a few days, it is not uncommon for some children to experience more serious local reactions. One reaction of this type, in which tissue becomes hardened or produces a hard nodule on the skin, is known as induration. Harris Coulter and Barbara Loe Fisher recount the extent of these nodules in their extraordinary book, DPT: A Shot in the Dark. One mother described the nodule on her infant son which developed about twenty-four hours after his DPT shot: He "had a knot about the size of a walnut or golf ball—it was red, hot, hard and really large—come up on his leg. It was there for about two months."[3] Another mother described the skin reaction caused by a DPT vaccine, which was "as big as the palm of my hand," and "swelled up like a giant hive" which covered the skin of her three-month-old infant girl.[4] This infant was left brain-damaged after her first DPT shot.

Systemic Reactions

Systemic reactions are ones that affect the entire body. The most common systemic reactions to the DPT vaccine, in no particular order are: vomiting, diarrhea, anorexia, cough, runny nose, and ear infections. Many of the children who react adversely to the DPT vaccine suffer allergies, colds, upper respiratory infections, and recurring ear infections for months or longer following one or more DPT shots.[5]

Neurological Reactions

While all reactions to the DPT vaccine are serious issues for parents, the vaccine is even more insidious in that it can produce damage, both temporary and permanent, to the central nervous system. Such reactions are known as neurological reactions.

Many bewildered and frightened parents have experienced the terror of seeing their once-healthy infants suffer a severe reaction to DPT just hours after an immunization shot. Two of the more common serious reactions, which have been witnessed by parents and physicians alike, are known as "high-pitched screaming" episodes and "persistent crying" spells. One mother describes the screaming bout of her infant son as a "blood-curdling scream like someone was stabbing him," after which the child became unresponsive and limp, only to repeat the whole process an hour later.[6] George Dick M.D., a British vaccine researcher, described the high-pitched screaming episode as lasting for an hour or more, after which the exhausted infant goes into a quiet period of about a half-hour, yet is still quite restless. The screaming pattern begins again, until the infant falls into a deep sleep, sometimes lasting up to twelve hours.[7]

The high-pitched screaming episodes and persistent crying bouts, while serious in themselves, are thought to be neurological warning signs of even greater brain dysfunction. In that regard, perhaps the most common serious reaction to the pertussis vaccine is the convulsive seizure.[8] One mother described her daughter's seizure following a DPT shot: "She would stare straight ahead with her eyes dilated and her mouth frozen open. Her lips were blue and her body stiff. The right side of her body would tremble and sometimes she would make sucking sounds while she was having the seizure."[9]

Another child reacted within seven hours of her first DPT shot with a high-pitched scream, rigid body, and staring look, followed by a sixteen-hour sleep.[10] Afterwards, her mother reported the reaction to her pediatrician. Upon seeing the child again, unbelievably, the physician proceeded to give the infant a second dose of DPT vaccine! Twelve hours later, the baby girl underwent a "tonic-clonic" convulsion lasting four and a half hours.[11] Thereafter, the vaccine-battered infant developed diarrhea, otitis media (middle ear infections), bronchial infections, runny nose, asthma, and an allergic reaction to all milk products.[12] The young child continues to have seizures, asthma, and "bouts" of pneumonia three years after her neurological shock with DPT vaccine.[13]

Infantile Spasms

Just about every form of seizure disorder, whether it is convulsions, epilepsy, grand mal, or petit mal, has been associated with the pertussis vaccine.[14] One powerful seizure disorder suffered in children less than two years old is known as infantile spasms or salaam seizures. The convulsive seizure is often described as a jack-knife seizure because the infant's head drops suddenly to its knees—or its knees come up to its chest.[15] When the seizure is accompanied by an abnormal EEG (brain wave pattern), suggestive of gross mental deficit, the name hypsarrythmia is given. It describes a convulsive seizure in which there is a sudden jerking of the head, the arms flinging upward, a general shaking in the body, and a "rolling up" of the eyes.[16]

In 1946, Douglas Buchanan, a Chicago-based neurologist, was one of the first physicians to bring this disorder to the attention of the medical profession. He believed that infantile spasms were being misdiagnosed in young children and that they were actually major convulsions. What is striking is that Buchanan began to observe infantile spasms in the mid-1940s when Evanston, Illinois, a nearby suburb, had one of the first and most extensive whooping cough vaccination clinics in the United States.[17] The type of convulsive seizure described by Buchanan was known as West's Syndrome prior to his observations, and only sixty-two cases were reported in the entire repertoire of medical literature between 1841 and 1948.[18] Between 1950 and 1963, however, at the same time DPT vaccinations were in full swing throughout the United States, 1,453 cases were reported.[19] By the 1970s, medical journals began filling with articles about infantile spasms seen in young children. Baird and Barofsky (1957), Jeavans and Bower (1964), Strom (1967), and Stewart (1979) had examined the issue of infantile spasms and concluded that pertussis vaccine was a distinct possibility as a cause—especially since the great majority of the infants, as often is the case, were healthy full-term babies, without an abnormal history prior to their DPT shot.

Before 1975, adverse reactions to vaccines were described as rare—both in medical journals and by the overwhelming majority of practicing pediatricians in America. Since the 1970s a number of comprehensive studies have been undertaken both in the United States and Great Britain to assess the frequency of reactions suffered in children following the administration of the DPT vaccine. What these studies illustrate, as you will quickly see, is that adverse reactions are not rare events—not by a long shot. Despite this, the medical profession has not only permitted the use of the DPT vaccine for the last fifty years, but has endorsed it—without ever knowing the rate of severe adverse reactions.

Table 10-1

PERCENT OF INFANTS AND CHILDREN SUFFERING ADVERSE REACTIONS TO DPT VACCINE, 1977-1978

TYPE OF REACTION	PERCENT
No Reaction	7.0
Mild	27.3
Moderate	58.6
Severe	7.1
Total Adverse Reactions	**93.0**

Based on 1,232 infants and children each receiving 5 DPT shots.
All adverse reactions occurring within 48 hours of inoculation.
Source: R.M. Barkin and M.E. Pichichero, "Diphtheria-Pertussis-Tetanus Vaccine: Reactogenicity of Commercial Products," *Pediatrics* 63, no. 2 (1979): 256-60.

DPT REACTIONS

The most revealing statistic is that 93 percent of all infants receiving the DPT vaccine had some sort of reaction to it—with over 65 percent of those reactions being moderate to severe (table 10-1). We also learn that of the 1,232 infants receiving five doses of DPT, 72 percent had a local reaction to the vaccine: pain, tenderness, redness, or swelling (table 10-2). In more prolonged local reactions, induration occurs—and some-times an abscess (granuloma) forms at the site of the injection.

The information in table 10-2 and 10-3 reveals that infants and children suffer systemic reactions, such as fever, vomiting, anorexia, and persistent crying spells in appreciable numbers following DPT inoculations. About half the children in both studies had a fever of over 100° with 81 percent experiencing some sort of behavioral change from the vaccine.

Table 10-2

LOCAL AND SYSTEMIC ADVERSE REACTIONS OCCURRING IN INFANTS AND CHILDREN FOLLOWING DPT VACCINE, 1977-1978

ADVERSE REACTION	PERCENT OF CHILDREN
NO LOCAL REACTION	27.8
LOCAL REACTIONS	
Redness	40.6
Swelling	37.8
Tenderness	52.4
TOTAL LOCAL REACTIONS	72.2
ACUTE BEHAVIORAL CHANGES	
No change	18.2
Irritable	33.8
Crying	35.1
Prolonged Screaming	12.9
TOTAL BEHAVIORAL CHANGES	81.8
FEVER	
<100 F	46.4
100 F - 102 F	49.4
>102 F	4.2

Based on 1,232 infants and children each receiving 5 DPT shots.
All adverse reactions occurring within 48 hours of inoculation.
Source: R.M.Barkin and M.E.Pichichero, "Diphtheria-Pertussis-Tetanus Vaccine: Reactogenicity of Commercial Products," *Pediatrics* 63, no. 2 (1979): 256-60.

Table 10-3

THE FDA-UCLA STUDY.
FREQUENCY OF SIMPLE, SYSTEMIC, AND NEUROLOGICAL ADVERSE REACTIONS FOLLOWING DPT VACCINE, 1981

REACTION[a]	PERCENT OF TOTAL DPT SHOTS
LOCAL REACTION	%
Redness	37.4
Swelling	40.7
Pain	50.9
SYSTEMIC REACTIONS	
Fever (>100.1 F)	46.5
Drowsiness	31.5
Anorexia	20.9
Persistent Crying	3.1
High-Pitched Screaming	.1
NEUROLOGICAL REACTIONS	NUMBER OBSERVED
Convulsions	9
Collapse[b]	9
Convulsions	1 per 1,750 doses
Collapse	1 per 1,750 doses

a. adverse reactions were calculated as a percentage of total DPT shots, whose aggregate number was 15,752.
b. hypotonic-hyporesponsive episodes
Source: C.L. Cody et al., "Nature and Rates of Adverse Reactions Associated with DTP and DT Immunization in Infants and Children," *Pediatrics* 68, no. 5 (1981): 650-60.

FREQUENCY OF NEUROLOGICAL REACTIONS

The FDA-UCLA study (table 10-3) measures the adverse reactions as a percentage of total immunization shots. At face value, it is difficult to gauge the results of this study, because the authors conveniently left out two crucial pieces of information: how many children were used in the vaccination survey and how many immunizations each child received. However, in an unpublished "Final Report" of the FDA-UCLA vaccine study prepared for the Bureau of Biologics, dated March 18, 1980, the number of children in the study was given as 16,536 on the title page and as "approximately 7,000 children" later on in the text.[20] Although we may never know the true number of participants, an excellent analysis of the data by Harris Coulter and Barbara Loe Fisher and a second analysis of the study done by Koplan and Hinman suggest that the 7,000 number is probably the closest to being accurate.[21]

The UCLA-FDA study reported nine convulsions and nine episodes of collapse. Because the published account in *Pediatrics* omitted crucial information, the results are misleading. According to this method, a convulsion occurred at the rate of 1 per every 1,750 DPT shots, as did the nine episodes of collapse. If you take these two neurological events together, there were eighteen neurological reactions following DPT immunization or a frequency of 1 per every 875 DPT shots. However, the previously mentioned unpublished "Final Report" revealed that there were about 7,000 children enrolled. If this is the case, then 1 in every 778 children suffered a convulsion from the vaccine, 1 in 778 children suffered a shock-collapse from the vaccine, or 1 in 389 children had some sort of neurological reaction to the vaccine (see table 10-4). Additionally, there were twenty-two cases of unusual crying (1 per 363 children), which the authors, unlike many other medical authorities, did not regard as a neurological reaction to the DPT vaccine.

In 1984, in their reanalysis of the FDA-UCLA vaccine study, Alan Hinman and Jeffrey Koplan estimate that there are 10,002 "complications" from DPT vaccine among one million children.[22] "Complications" were defined as convulsions, collapse, and high-pitched screaming episodes. If about 3.3 million children are vaccinated for DPT each year in the U.S., than some 33,006 children (10,002 x 3.3) are suffering adverse neurological damage each year (see table 10-5). It is not hard for me to believe that this large number of babies are seriously hurt each year from taking DPT vaccine when you consider that adverse reactions, debilitating conditions, and diseases have

Table 10-4

THE FREQUENCY OF NEUROLOGICAL REACTIONS FOLLOWING DPT IMMUNIZATIONS BASED ON 7,000 INFANTS AND CHILDREN ENROLLED IN THE UCLA-FDA STUDY

REACTION	NUMBER OF CHILDREN HAVING A REACTION	FREQUENCY
Convulsions	9	1 in every 778 children
Shock-Collapse	9	1 in every 778 children
Serious Neurological Reaction	18	1 in every 389 children
Unusual Crying	22	1 in every 363 children

Source: Pertussis Vaccine Project: *Rates, Nature and Etiology of Adverse Reactions Associated with DTP Vaccine.* Prepared for the Bureau of Biologics, Food and Drug Administration, March 18,1980. Cited in H. Coulter and B.L. Fisher, *DPT: A Shot in the Dark* (New York, Harcourt Brace Jovanovich, 1985), pp. 243-48.

Table 10-5

AN ESTIMATE OF TOTAL ACUTE NEUROLOGICAL REACTIONS TO THE DPT VACCINE IN THE UNITED STATES EACH YEAR, 1984

Number of children immunized each year for DPT vaccine	3,300,000
Number of children having convulsions	8,484
Number of children having a collapse	8,484
Number of children having high-pitched screaming episodes	16,038
Annual total of acute neurological reactions	33,006

A reanalysis of the UCLA-FDA study of 1979 (modified).
Source: Alan Hinman and Jeffrey Koplan, "Pertussis and Pertussis Vaccine: Reanalysis of Benefits, Risks, and Costs," *Journal of the American Medical Association* 251, no. 23 (1984): 3109-13.

Table 10-6

DEATHS FROM DPT VACCINE

Number of U.S. children receiving DPT Vaccine each year	3,300,000
Number of deaths in UCLA-FDA study	2
Rate of deaths using 7,000 infants enrolled in study	1 per 3,500 children
Annual total of children killed in the U.S. by DPT vaccine	943

Source: H. Coulter and B.L. Fisher, *DPT: A Shot in the Dark* (New York: Harcourt Brace Jovanovich, 1985), p.374.

followed the use of diphtheria, pertussis, and tetanus vaccines since 1900 (see table 10-7).

Vaccine reactions, syndromes, and vaccine-related deaths happen every day in the United States—and all over the world. On July 3, 1991, the National Academy of Science's Institute of Medicine released a report, "Adverse Effects of Pertussis and Rubella Vaccines."[61] This report was the result of a twenty-month review of the medical literature and was requested by Congress as part of the National Childhood Vaccine Injury Act of 1986. In its report the DPT vaccine was "indicated" as a cause of acute brain injury, anaphylactic shock, shock-collapse, inconsolable crying, and febrile seizures.[62] The rubella vaccine

Table 10-7

REACTIONS, SYNDROMES, DISEASES, AND DEATHS
FOLLOWING DIPHTHERIA, PERTUSSIS AND
TETANUS VACCINES, 1900-1983

VACCINE	YEAR	ADVERSE REACTION
Diphtheria antiserum	1901	tetanus, 20 cases, 14 deaths [23]
Diphtheria toxin-antitoxin mixture (TAM)	1919	diphtheria intoxication, 120 cases, 10 deaths skin eruptions, acute lymphangitis, fever, nausea, vomiting, neuromuscular paralysis, death [24]
Tetanus and diphtheria antiserums	1932	serum neuritis, polyneuritis [25, 26]
Pertussis vaccine	1933	convulsions, sudden death [27]
Diphtheria antiserum	1942	serum sickness, fever, edema, adenopathy, arthritis, myositis [28]
Alum precipitated pertussis vaccine	1945	abscess formation [29]
Tetanus toxoid	1945	hepatitis [30]
Diphtheria toxoid Pertussis antigen	1946	anaphylactic shock, death [31]
Pertussis vaccine	1948	severe encephalopathy, chronic convulsions, comatose state, severe mental retardation, cerebral palsy, blindness, death [32]

Table 10-7, continued

VACCINE	YEAR	ADVERSE REACTION
Alum-precipitated toxoid	1948	edema, heart failure, paralysis, ulceration, death 606 cases, 68 deaths [33]
Pertussis vaccine	1949	encephalopathy, death [34]
Pertussis vaccine	1949	fever, convulsions, death [35]
DPT	1949-1953	fever, convulsions, irreversible brain damage, death [36]
Diphtheria-pertussis vaccine	1953	poliomyelitis provoked by DP vaccine [37]
Antitetanus serum	1954	radiculitis, polyneuritis, Guillain-Barré syndrome, optic neuritis, Landry's paralysis, myelitis [38]
Diphtheria-pertussis	1954	screaming, drowsiness, convulsions, vomiting, myoclonic twitching [39]
Diphtheria	1954	transverse myelitis [40]
DPT	1955-1961	mental retardation, cerebral palsy, recurrent convulsions 22 cases in institutions [41]
DPT	1961-1972	neurological reactions, paralysis, mental retardation, epilepsy, death [42]
DPT	1977	marble pallor, interrupted sleep, paralysis, refusal of food, convulsions, subnormal mentality, hyperactivity, infantile spasms, epilepsy, unresponsiveness to parents [43]

Table 10-7, continued

VACCINE	YEAR	ADVERSE REACTION
DPT	1978	convulsions, infantile spasms, persistent screaming, collapse, encephalopathy, cardiac arrest, residual brain damage, Reye's syndrome, death [44]
DPT	1979	bulging fontanelle (increased intra-cranial pressure) [45]
DPT	1979	screaming attacks, convulsions, collapse, spasticity, paralysis, hyperactivity, epilepsy, convulsions, 197 cases [46]
DPT	1982	sudden infant death syndrome [47]

The citations used in table 10-7 were drawn from articles published in medical journals during the last eighty-five years. The articles document the adverse events that have followed the use of diphtheria, pertussis, and tetanus vaccines. In general, the adverse vaccine reaction occurred within 2 to 25 days following the inoculation. However, many adverse reactions occur within hours of inoculation. Historically, adverse reactions have followed the use of all vaccines and serums including: yellow fever, typhoid, hepatitis, BCG, mumps, measles, rubella, smallpox, polio, and influenza. See table 10-8 for a small sampling of adverse events that have occurred after vaccinations.

was also indicated as having a causal link to chronic arthritis in women.[63]

The National Childhood Vaccine Injury Act of 1986 (PL 99-660) was signed into law as a no-fault compensation program for people who were killed or permanently injured as a result of receiving one or more of the currently mandated vaccines: measles, mumps, rubella, diphtheria, pertussis, tetanus, and polio. In order to qualify for monetary compensation, a person

Table 10-8

Disease Following Vaccinations

Type of Vaccine	Disease
1. Live rubella	arthritis [48]
2. Smallpox, yellow fever, typhoid, rabies, TB	multiple sclerosis [49]
3. Yellow fever	jaundice [50, 51]
4. Live measles	learning disabilities, profound mental retardation, hemiparesis, cerebral palsy [52]
5. Mumps convalescent serum	hepatitis [53]
6. Hemophilus influenzae type B	meningitis [54]
7. DPT	paralytic polio [55, 56]
8. Smallpox	post-vaccinal encephalitis and death [57, 58]
9. Measles vaccine (attenuated)	middle ear infections, tonsillitis, convulsions, delirium [59]
10. Diphtheria-tetanus toxoid, oral polio vaccine	tinnitus, permanent deafness [60]

must have injuries that persisted for six months or more and cost at least $1000 in out-of-pocket expenses.[64]

As of February 1992 a total of 353 awards totaling $202.5 million had been awarded to individuals who were either injured or killed by a vaccine.[65] A profile of 3,176 vaccine compensation cases submitted to the U.S. Claims Court and abstracted

Table 10-9

VACCINE INJURY COMPENSATION PROGRAM
SUMMARY OF 3,176 CASES ABSTRACTED
FEBRUARY 18, 1992[1]

VACCINES LISTED IN PETITIONS:

Vaccine	Total	Injury	Death
DT [a]	21	16	5
DTP [b]	2272	1862	410
Pertussis	2	0	2
Tetanus	2	2	0
IPV/OPV*	11	10	1
IPV [c]	242	232	10
OPV [d]	196	181	15
MMR [e]	178	164	14
Measles	90	78	12
Mumps	8	8	0
Rubella	102	101	1
Non-qualified**	24	22	2
Unspecified*	28	27	1
Totals	**3,176**	**2,703**	**473**

1. From 1988 to 1992
*Insufficient information submitted to make determination
**Vaccines not covered
(Represents only a partial listing of total cases filed and interpretation of the data should be cautious)

a. Diphtheria/Tetanus toxoid (combined)
b. Diphtheria/Tetanus toxoid and pertussis (combined)
c. Inactivated polio vaccine
d. Oral polio vaccine
e. Measles/Mumps/Rubella (combined)

Source: Department of Health and Human Services, Public Health Service, Bureau of Health Professions, Health Resources and Services Administration, Rockville, Maryland.

by the Vaccine Injury Compensation Program is given in table 10-9.

There were 2,703 injuries and 473 deaths from childhood vaccines abstracted from these claims. Every one of the current childhood vaccines has caused either injury or death to infants and children. The theoretical assumption behind the alleged success of immunization is that a carefully controlled amount of antigen is used in the vaccine, enough to stimulate immunity yet not enough to cause disease or death. We now know with certainty that, while the concept looks good on paper, in real life it is a myth.

CHAPTER 11

Measles in the 1980s

*T*he mysteries of vaccination and the promotion of its alleged value in protecting children from disease and reducing disease transmission can no better be seen for what they are than in the current situation with measles. Since 1983, large outbreaks of measles have continued to occur in the United States at an increasing rate. As of May 1991, an unofficial total of 27,672 cases had been reported in the United States for 1990.[1] This represented a large increase from 1989, when 18,193 cases were reported and was the single highest total since 1978.[2] What is perplexing to many epidemiologists and downright embarrassing to some is that most cases of measles in 1989 occurred in two distinct populations: children less than sixteen months who are primarily unvaccinated; and adolescent, high school, and college age students, ages ten to nineteen, of whom 90 percent or more are vaccinated.[3]

It is predictable, though not acceptable, that infants less than sixteen months old, who are most susceptible, can suffer severely from measles. But for adolescents, high school age children, and even college students to develop measles is not expected, especially since the overwhelming majority have been vaccinated. In order to understand why measles has increased so dramatically in older age groups, a number of important factors will be considered. These include: measles in the pre-vaccine era, the age at which children are immunized for measles, the negative immune response to the measles vaccine, the role of measles vaccine during epidemics, and severe syndromes that have resulted from the vaccine.

Measles Before the Vaccine

Measles is an acute infectious disease of childhood, marked first by its small bluish-red spots (known as Koplik spots) on the skin and later by a rash. It is usually accompanied by fever, hacking cough, conjunctivitis, nasal discharge, watery eyes (coryza), and intolerance to light (photophobia). Despite its prevalence in the United States in the decades preceding the measles vaccines, measles was a self-limiting illness with a low mortality, and was benign in the greatest majority of children.[4] During the years from 1950 to 1962, in what has become known as the pre-measles vaccine era, there were about 500,000 reported cases of measles each year in the United States.[5] Of all the people who contracted measles during these years, more than 50 percent were children between the ages of five and nine.[6] In fact, about 95 percent of naturally acquired measles was in children less than fifteen years old.[7] For at least four decades before the introduction of the measles vaccine in 1963, measles epidemics occurred at regular intervals, every two or three years. Seasonally, measles peaked during the spring months, from March to June, and declined in late summer and fall, August to November. After the measles vaccine was introduced, a number of significant changes took place. One of these is the age at which children are now becoming infected with the wild measles virus caught naturally from exposure.

The Use of Live and Killed Vaccines

In March 1963, two different measles vaccines became available to the American public: the attenuated "live" measles vaccine, known as the Edmonston B vaccine, and the inactivated "killed" vaccine, which used alum as a preservative and formalin to inactivate the measles virus. The "killed" measles vaccine was used in the U.S. from 1963 to 1967. It is estimated that about 1.8 million doses of the vaccine were produced and distributed to between 600,000 and 900,000 children.[8] From 1963 to 1976, 88 million doses of "live" measles vaccine were distributed in the United States; 19 million doses were Edmonston B vaccine, and 69 million were further attenuated strains.[9]

Between 1971 and 1975, when measles vaccination programs were in full swing in the United States and about 69 percent of children ages one to thirteen were vaccinated against measles, the number of reported cases of measles diminished in the traditionally active five-to-nine age group, from greater than 50 percent (during the 1950s) to about 31 percent in 1975.[10] Moreover, the rate of measles increased significantly in adolescents older than fifteen, from about 5 percent (during the 1950s) to 14 percent during the years 1971 to 1975.[11] During the 1980s, as vaccination quotas averaged better than 90 percent for school children, measles infiltrated a wide variety of age groups, including infants less than one, adolescents older than fifteen, college age students, and adults over twenty-five.

By 1989, with over 98 percent of school-age children immunized against measles by the time they entered the first grade,[12] only 10 per cent of all reported cases of measles occurred in children aged five to nine.[13] This age range is by far the most likely time a child would contract natural measles infection before there was a vaccine. By contrast, 41 per cent of all reported cases of measles in 1989 occurred in people fifteen years or older; 8 per cent of these were in people twenty-five years or older, largely an unknown category of measles sufferers in the 1950s.[14]

This phenomenon has not been adequately explained by the medical profession, nor, as my research has uncovered, has it even been given great significance. It is my belief, however, that the appearance of measles in older age groups is indeed serious—and is related, in one way or another, to the measles vaccine.

Measles In Highly Vaccinated Children, Adolescents, and College Students

The United States Immunization Survey of 1981 revealed that 77 percent of individuals aged five to nineteen had received mumps vaccine, 85 percent rubella vaccine, and 86 percent measles vaccine.[15] During the 1988-89 school year, more than 98 percent of school children were vaccinated against pertussis, measles, mumps, rubella, and polio, by the time they entered the first grade.[16]

Since 1983, a copious number of articles and reports have appeared in medical journals and in *Morbidity and Mortality Weekly Report*, (Centers for Disease Control) documenting measles outbreaks in highly vaccinated school-age populations and in adults over the age of twenty. In 1989, there were 248 outbreaks in the United States, of which 170 occurred in children ages five to nineteen, 56 in pre-schoolers less than five, and 22 in post-school-age adults, twenty years or older.[17] Between 1983 and 1985 there were more than a dozen reported outbreaks of measles in Texas among junior and senior high school students of whom 95 percent had received measles vaccine, as confirmed by school immunization records.[18]

In 1985, a measles outbreak among students in Corpus Christi, Texas, demonstrated that 99 percent of the students had valid proof of measles immunization.[19] When blood samples were taken from 1,806 students one week after the first case surfaced, they revealed that more than 95 percent of those tested were considered "immune" to measles; this was confirmed by a sophisticated test called enzyme-linked immunosorbent assay or ELISA.[20] This means that 95 percent of the students tested, of whom 99 percent were adequately immunized, had detectable antibody in their blood to measles, the standard by which immunity is gauged. Furthermore, 12 percent of the students in Corpus Christi had received two doses of measles vaccine.[21] Despite all the "scientific" proofs that these children were immune to measles, epidemics broke out among highly vaccinated students nonetheless.

In 1989, a measles epidemic occurred in Chicago, affecting some 2,232 people. Afro-Americans suffered 1,594 cases (71 percent), Hispanics accounted for 506 cases (23 percent), and the remaining 6 percent occurred in Caucasians and other groups.[22] Whereas the Texas outbreaks affected highly vaccinated adolescents, the Chicago epidemic occurred primarily in unvaccinated infants and children, 75 percent of whom were less than five years of age. What made this particular epidemic noteworthy is that 32 percent of the measles cases occurred in infants less than fifteen months old, or below the minimum age for measles vaccine.

That children under the age of fifteen months can develop measles certainly is not a new phenomenon; its historical pattern has been established for at least the last seventy years. The point I wish to consider (and it is crucial) is how the Chicago Health Department dealt with the problem, which was by lowering the minimum age for measles vaccination to twelve months—and later to six months. Before we can see the effect of lowering the minimum age for vaccination in Chicago in 1989, we need to take a brief retrospective look at some important points about measles vaccine during the last thirty years.

At What Age Should a Child Receive a Vaccine?

Historically, the age at which vaccines are given to infants and children has varied considerably. In England, the DPT vaccine or "triple vaccine" is administered at six months, while in the United States infants begin DPT shots, as well as polio shots, at two months.

The ages at which vaccines are "recommended" by the experts follow some general guidelines, yet ones that are easily violated. Again, using the antibody response as a yardstick, one criterion used for determining the magic age for measles inoculation is the age at which 95 percent of infants uniformly produce detectable antibody to the measles vaccine.[23] In 1963, the year measles vaccine was introduced, the recommended age was nine months.[24] The thinking at that time was that maternal antibodies waned at about seven months. In 1965, the recommended age was raised to twelve months after new data revealed that maternal antibodies persist in the infant until eleven months.[25] However, in 1977, the Committee on Infectious Diseases of the American Academy of Pediatrics and the Public Health Service Advisory Committee on Immunization Practices recommended that infants receive the vaccine at fifteen months, after discovering that infants at twelve months of age have lower rates of "seropositivity," the rate at which measles vaccines produce antibodies in the infants, than infants at fourteen months of age.[26] Additionally, to complicate matters further, in 1973, an article appearing in the *Journal of the American Medical Association* entitled "Neurologic Disorders Following Live Measles-Virus Vaccination," revealed that in 1963 and 1964, the average age reported to the Centers for Disease Control for neurological reactions within thirty days of a live measles vaccine was seven years old.[27] It appears that, in the early days of measles vaccination, seven-year-old children were getting the vaccine, even though the recommended age was nine months! Furthermore, during the first few years after the vaccine was licensed, children were getting three doses of measles vaccine at one month intervals, and in some cases, were receiving two doses of killed vaccine and one dose of live vaccine.[28]

One major reason that there is a minimum age for vaccination is that if an infant receives a vaccine at too early an age, the vaccine interferes with maternal antibodies already in place, which were passed from mother to fetus in the blood circulation. The presence of maternal antibodies may depress or alter the infant's immune response to the vaccine antigen. According to the *Merck Manual*, infants have a "deficient" response to certain vaccine antigens to begin with, and if immunization shots begin too early, "it may result in the development of a tolerance or a decreased antibody response to subsequent challenge with the same antigen."[29] Even more specifically, there is about a "five-fold or greater" chance of an infant contracting measles if it is vaccinated before fifteen months.[30] Walter Orenstein, M.D., and associates who studied the effects of revaccinating for measles children who had received primary measles vaccine before ten months of age, revealed that not only did the infants have an "altered" immune reaction to the vaccine antigen from the first measles shot, but that they may have a similar abortive response when they are revaccinated as older children.[31] With these observations in mind the actions taken by the Chicago Health Department are quite disturbing.

Measles in Chicago

The measles outbreak in Chicago began on February 14, 1989. From this day forward, until the time the minimum age for measles vaccine was lowered to twelve months on May 5, 1989, cases of measles continued to climb. The number of cases reached a peak in July 1989.[32] Thus, vaccinating children under the age of fifteen months while the epidemic was occurring apparently had no effect on reducing measles transmission, thereby failing to reduce the measles caseload. Furthermore, and equally unconscionable, the health department lowered the minimum age a second time on July 31, 1989 to six months of age for infants in high-risk areas. Over the next couple of months this was accompanied by intense door-to-door surveillance by the health department to educate and vaccinate inner-city residents of housing projects. During the epidemic, cases of measles began to decline during the months of July down through November, especially in the months of August, September, and October, when cases of measles are traditionally and seasonally at their lowest.[33] The rise in measles cases that occurred from March to June coincided exactly with the months when measles is historically most prevalent in the United States, and has been for the last sixty years or more.[34] In addition, from 1947 to 1967, measles epidemics of varying intensities have consistently occurred in Chicago about every two years, both before and after measles vaccine was introduced.[35]

Because of these historical factors, which substantiate a pattern for measles transmission that transcends man's abortive attempts to artificially control measles by mass inoculation, I seriously doubt that lowering the minimum measles age, from fifteen months to twelve months and then finally to six months for high-risk children, did anything to stop the transmission of measles or protect susceptible infants from contracting measles. In 1967, twenty-two years earlier, Chicago had suffered a similar measles epidemic and tried to solve the problem the same way it tried to solve the 1989 one, by immunizing people with measles vaccine during the epidemic.[36] The frenetic measles inoculation program, which was covered in the *Journal of the American Medical Association,* failed to terminate or alter the epidemic.[37]

These examples provide strong evidence that measles vaccines given during epidemics fail to control the epidemic. The continued practice of immunizing children during epidemics shows clearly that health departments believe undyingly in immunization, despite evidence that it is a poor protector of infants' and children's health. In fact, it appears that the only way health departments can deal with any outbreak of childhood illness is to vaccinate and vaccinate again. This is done at the incredible risk of injuring an infant's immune response, one of the most vital immunological functions. This is not good medicine, but, rather, medical fanaticism at its worst.

Susceptibility To Measles

In order to gain an understanding of why some infants are so susceptible to measles, even today, it is useful to look to the past for important clues.

In 1899, in the worst of times at the Infants and Children's Hospital on Randall's Island in New York City, 107 children, who were currently hospitalized for measles, were observed. Sixty-two of the children had other complicating medical conditions, such as tuberculosis, enteritis, broncho-pneumonia, bronchitis, diphtheria, and scarlet fever.[38]   Of the twenty children who apparently died from measles, fourteen deaths (70 percent) were attributed to other causes.[39]   It may be that measles was the infection that overwhelmed these unfortunate children and took them over the edge to death; nonetheless the greatest majority already suffered from some other debilitating condition.

It has been noted earlier, from reports of the White House Conference on Child Health in 1930, that high fatality rates from measles in infant asylums during the 1920s were caused by unusual risk factors that may have enhanced measles deaths. These included malnutrition, overcrowding, inadequate nursing care, and poor hygiene.[40] It was also noted that the high number of fatalities among Blacks and Native Americans during this time was more likely due to living conditions than to any increased susceptibility because of race or other inherent qualities.[41]

The team of physician-researchers who investigated the Chicago measles epidemic of 1967 discovered that most cases of measles occurred in the lowest socio-economic areas of Chicago.[42] During other measles outbreaks that arose throughout the United States in 1989, measles occurred in increasing numbers in Black and Hispanic preschool children living in the inner-city. We are told by the CDC that many of these children are undervaccinated. Again, they suggest, as usual, that this may be the reason for the increase in measles cases.[43] However, I assert that the alleged undervaccination is not the problem— nor even a problem. The U.S. Immunization Survey of 1987 (unpublished CDC) revealed that 82 percent of preschool children in the United States had been vaccinated for measles by their second birthday.[44] Even more recent information concerning the vaccination status of preschool children in inner-city schools in eight large cities in the United States for 1989 demonstrated that 69 percent of the children had been vaccinated for measles and that 63 percent of Black and Hispanic children were vaccinated for measles by their second birthday.[45] Of course, by the time these children reach kindergarten, because of mandatory state immunization laws, about 98 per cent will have been vaccinated. Even if undervaccination were the problem, these high numbers of preschool vaccinated children would not substantiate the "undervaccinated" argument. Again, since it has been demonstrated that both vaccinated and unvaccinated children get measles, to say that undervaccination is the cause is weak. It is more likely that these Black and Hispanic preschool children, like the people in the Chicago measles epidemic of 1967, were the product of low-income families receiving inadequate heath care and nutrition. If some of these children are malnourished, receiving inadequate parental care, or living in overcrowded, deteriorating environments or if they have some other underlying health condition that would put them at special risk, then they will be much more likely to suffer severe complications from measles, and perhaps even die. Unfortunately

I do not have more specific information on the living arrangements, family situation, or individual health profiles for the children. Historically, however, as I have shown, measles deaths have been the result of overcrowding, malnutrition, deficient hygiene and heath care, and occasioned by underlying health conditions. Edward Godfrey, who investigated measles in infant asylums during the 1920s, said this about the illness: "The causes of a high fatality rate in measles are usually, if not always, in the physical condition of the patient, faults in his [her] environment or care for the sick—rarely—if ever, in an inherent virulence of the disease itself."[46]

In 1989 there were forty-one "measles associated" deaths among 18,183 reported measles cases in the United States.[47] The fact that they are called "measles associated" deaths suggests involvement with other conditions. In 1989, according to the CDC, about 30 percent of those suffering measles associated deaths between the ages of nineteen and thirty-five years old had a pre-existing medical condition such as diabetes, leukemia, or scleroderma.[48] Of the thirty-one measles associated deaths that occurred in infants and children less than five years old in 1989, of whom twenty-nine we are told were unvaccinated, at least two children had pre-existing medical conditions, (leukemia and congenital neurological defects); one case occurred in a vaccinated child, the other in a unvaccinated child.[49] Nine deaths occurred in infants less than one year old, in whom vaccination was not yet indicated.

What conclusions can be drawn from all this? That infants and children die from measles or from pneumonia occasioned by measles is a sad fact of life. Thirty-one children under the age of five dying, while never acceptable, is a miniscule number compared to the thousands of infants who die each year from sudden infant death syndrome or from accidents in the home. What seems to get lost amidst the irrational fear of the pro-vaccination zealots is that measles is a self-limiting illness, rarely fatal in a healthy child.

Perhaps this is the most sobering fact about measles, mumps, rubella, and even polio. None are particularly fatal diseases in healthy children. Even diphtheria and whooping cough, which conjure up memories of fear and death among older Americans, declined in mortality more than 70 percent from 1885 to 1935. This pattern was well established decades before mass immunization programs began on a large scale. And yet a very small percentage of children are particularly susceptible to all these childhood diseases, in the sense of suffering death or lingering conditions from them. The reason, perhaps, is that they are malnourished, live in crowded unhygienic circumstances, or suffer from some other underlying medical condition. The healthy baby or child can withstand an attack of measles and becomes stronger because of it. The sickly baby suffers the severe consequences of measles, perhaps because its immune system cannot overcome the increased burden of infection.

Atypical Measles Syndrome

Along with unvaccinated infants and highly vaccinated school age children, all of whom contract measles, it has been established that an unknown number of children who were vaccinated with killed measles vaccines between 1963 and 1967, and even with some live measles vaccines which were damaged during storage, developed a condition known as atypical measles syndrome (AMS). The disease is characterized by high fever, toxicity, abdominal pain, and cough.[50] A rash occurs one or two days later and can be accompanied by edema of the hands and feet, pneumonia, glandular disease, and "nodular densities" in the lungs resulting in oxygen deficiency in the blood. Vincent Fulginiti, M.D., who along with associates investigated at least ten cases of atypical measles syndrome in 1967 suggests that these children's response to the "wild" measles virus is "altered."[51] He notes that other symptoms of the disease such as the "severity and persistence" of headache, when present, (and presumably much more severe than in natural measles), suggests "central nervous system" involvement, meaning encephalopathy (brain damage). Atypical measles syndrome has been definitively linked to the killed measles vaccine used in the U.S. from 1963 to 1967.[52] In 1967, Fulginiti, who once served as chairman of the American Academy of Pediatrics Committee on Infectious

Diseases, asserted that inactivated measles virus vaccine should no longer be administered.[53] Since 1967, the killed measles vaccine has no longer been used in the United States because of the untold health damage it caused, in the form of atypical measles syndrome. "We suspect that the reported cases [of atypical measles] represent a fraction of the total number that occur."[54] A more candid statement of unreported vaccine failures may never be uttered again from the lips of ardent vaccinators.

Neurological Reactions to the Measles Vaccine

From 1963 to 1971, eighty-four neurological reactions to the live measles vaccine were reported in the United States, the majority of cases clustering six to fifteen days following the injection.[55] Like the cases of AMS, these eighty-four neurological reactions are undoubtedly only a fraction of the actual total. Among the children who suffered needlessly, five died from "overwhelming" bacterial or viral infection. The post-mortem examination revealed pneumonitis in all five.[56] Eleven other children suffered from febrile convulsions. When follow-up work was done on eight of these children, all had recovered from their seizure disorders. Others were not so lucky. Fifty-nine children had "extensive neurological disorders" including encephalomyelitis (inflammation of the brain and spinal cord), ataxia (defective muscular control, resulting in jerky movements) and transverse myelitis (an acute inflammation of both sides of the spinal cord). When follow-up work was initiated on thirty-one children who suffered encephalopathies (brain damage), sixteen were found to have permanent neurological disorders such as aseptic meningitis, cranial nerve palsy, learning disabilities, hyperkinesis, and severe mental retardation.[57]

Immune Serum Globulin

Since 1963, untold numbers of children suffered syndromes and neurological disorders within a matter of days following inoculation with measles vaccine. Additional evidence has demonstrated that measles immune serum globulin (ISG) used in thousands of children since the 1930s may also have delayed or altered measles expression to adolescent or adult years or produced a wide variety of debilitating conditions in the wake of its use. In a reliable study done in Denmark in 1985 and reported in the medical journal *Lancet*, a significantly greater number of people who did not have measles as children, but showed specific IgG measles antibody in their blood as adults, were shown to subsequently suffer from immunoreactive diseases, sebaceous skin diseases, tumors, and degenerative diseases of bone and cartilage, than a matched control group, all of whom had measles as children.[58]

The study compared two groups of adults from Copenhagen and Gentofte, Denmark, all of whom were born in the 1940s. Among fifty-six adults who showed no history of measles, fifty-three (95 percent) had specific IgG measles antibody in their blood, the indicator of prior infection with measles virus. In the control group, among fifty-nine individuals who had measles as children, all showed evidence of specific IgG antibody in their blood.[59] In the non-measles group, it was confirmed that measles infection had taken place when the subjects were children, yet without the usual measles rash. The rash or spots that appear on the skin during measles are the places where the body literally "incinerates" the measles virus through cell-mediated reactions.[60] Thirteen individuals in the non-measles group presented evidence that they were given immune serum globulin as children after being exposed to measles. In this group, chondromalacia, a form of osteoarthritis affecting the cartilage, usually with pain and stiffness to joints, was observed in three subjects. In two of the individuals, the immune serum globulin was given when they were infants; chondromalacia was diagnosed in both at age seventeen.[61] In the third case, the individual was administered ISG at age nine, after being exposed to measles, and subsequently was diagnosed for chondromalacia at age thirty-six.[62] Other diseases that occurred in the individuals who were given immune serum globulin as children were: lupus erythematosus, a chronic condition affecting the skin, which the medical profession still regards as a disease of unknown origin, and Scheuermann's disease, another somewhat common disease affecting adolescents and characterized by lower back pain and excessive curvature of the spine, presumably from changes in the vertebrae.

Among the entire group of people whose school records and own verbal testimony corroborated that measles was absent in childhood (no rash), though evidence of measles antibody as adults revealed otherwise, there was an increased risk of 20 percent for four categories of diseases: sebaceous skin diseases, degenerative diseases of bone and cartilage, immunoreactive diseases, and tumors.[63] Some of the individual disease conditions were: lupus erythematosus; thyroiditis; arthralgia; Crohn's disease; orchitis; dermatitis-eczema; severe acne; alopecia; folliculitis; anal fistula; tibial fibroma; tumors of the vocal cords; sublingual, labial, and vaginal cysts; blast cell leukemia; carcinoma of the uterus and testis; and Scheuermann's disease. In the group of people who had measles as children, certainly there were cases of miscellaneous skin diseases, some immunoreactive disease, and atopic diseases. The author of the study, Tove Ronne, postulates that the presence of measles-virus-specific antibodies at the time of infection interferes with the body's immunological response to measles, especially with cell-mediated immunity, allowing measles virus to survive within the cells, causing disease in adulthood. It was the high number of disease conditions in the group of adults who exhibited no measles rash as children that prompted the authors to conclude that there is a "highly significant association" between the missed measles rash in childhood and the development of the aforementioned disease conditions later in life.[64]

Measles in College Settings

Because so many cases of measles have been occurring since 1983, in previously vaccinated high-school and college age students and in young adults ages twenty to twenty-five, the Immunization Practices Advisory Committee, as of 1989, now recommends two doses of measles vaccine.[65] The American College Health Association has taken a stand on the measles problem by recommending that colleges and universities adopt a policy that would make college students responsible for providing evidence that they are immune to measles and other so-called "vaccine preventable" diseases.[66] If that were not enough, the students must do this or face the threat of not being allowed to matriculate.[67] Since 1990, these policies or "laws" have been implemented by colleges and universities in twenty-two states, as well as the District of Columbia and Puerto Rico and are known as the Prematriculation Immunization Requirement.[68]

One way colleges and universities are enforcing this outrageous policy is by requiring students to provide evidence of two measles shots.[69] Since the Immunization Practices Advisory Committee (1989) only recently changed its tune from recommending one measles shot to two, this means that most college students in twenty-two states must submit to a second measles shot, or they can't enroll in school. Students also have the option of providing evidence that they previously had natural measles (physician-diagnosed cases) or "laboratory evidence" that they are immune to measles. Based on what we've discussed so far about measles, these requirements are laughable. Suffice it to say, however, that if college students are not savvy enough to exercise their individual right to oppose immunization on religious, medical, or philosophical grounds, which is still the only legal way to oppose immunizations, they'll be rolling up their sleeves for a painful and unnecessary measles shot, and all that it implies.

There is no evidence that getting two measles shots will prevent or contain measles. How could it? If one shot didn't work, what makes anyone think that two will? On the contrary, in 1985, in a study appearing in *Pediatrics* entitled "Risk Factors for Measles Vaccine Failure Among Immunized Students," 6.5 percent of students who became sick with measles had been vaccinated twice.[70] During the measles outbreak in Corpus Christi, Texas, in 1985, where 99 percent of the students were vaccinated against measles and 95 percent were considered immune by ELISA testing, 12 percent of the students had received two doses of measles vaccine to no avail.[71] Again, where's the protection?

The recent requirement making college students get additional measles shots (or two shots of any vaccine) is just one more flagrant example of the blind leading the blind. What makes this college immunization requirement particularly loathsome, like the mandatory immunization requirement for all American school children, is that it puts enormous pressure on parents and students to comply— or suffer the consequences. The vast majority of students don't know about religious or personal belief exemptions to immunization, primarily because information of this kind is not advertised, nor does the medical profession or the schools typically inform students of their rightful legal choice in the matter. Students who do not want to be immunized are thus clearly disadvantaged.

I hope that college students who in any way question or oppose immunizations will have enough self-respect and gumption to challenge this oppressive school requirement by exercising their individual right to oppose all immunizations on either medical, religious, or philosophical grounds, and by organizing themselves in demanding that the Prematriculation Immunization Requirement be repealed.

The Consequences of Measles Suppression

In the decade before the measles vaccines were introduced in the U.S. in 1963, natural measles infection occurred in great numbers of U.S. school children, perhaps as high as 80 percent or more. The greatest majority of cases occurred in children ages five to nine, and the rest in adolescents under the age of fifteen. After 1963, measles began to shift to older age groups and by the 1980s a significant number of people from infants less than age one to adults aged nineteen to thirty-five were contracting measles. I believe that the shift in measles infection to older age groups was caused by measles vaccines.

The primary negative effect of the vaccine has been in distorting the immune response of infants. We have seen that infants who became immunized before ten months of age during the 1960s had a five-fold greater chance of developing measles later on as children or adolescents. We have also witnessed that the killed measles vaccine and some live measles vaccines produced a new disease in an unknown number of children, called atypical measles syndrome. Some of the children who received these vaccines failed to be protected from future bouts of measles; some suffered brain damage, and others developed a new, more serious disease syndrome in the process.

In the case of children who received immune serum globulin after they were exposed to measles, the antibodies in the serum perhaps interfered with the immunological response to the "wild" measles virus incubating in the child. The immune serum globulin may have altered measles expression or delayed it to a later date. One result is that children may have experienced measles infection without the usual rash. Thus, the disease is hardly recognizable as measles, if it lacks its most recognizable symptom. Because measles was denied its natural expression of a skin rash, the virus remained inside human cells only to reappear later in life as grave skin diseases, cancer, arthritis, tumors, and disease syndromes affecting bone and cartilage.

The Centers for Disease Control report that 40 percent of all cases of measles in 1989 were in vaccinated individuals or could be attributed to "primary measles vaccine failure."[72] The same percentages of vaccine failure were given for fourteen investigated measles outbreaks that occurred in 1977 (table 11-1). I suspect that the number of measles cases occurring in vaccinated individuals during the last fifteen years has actually been higher than the 40 percent figure cited by the CDC, especially since about 90 percent of the population between the ages of five and thirty-five is currently vaccinated for measles. In any event, the 40 percent figure is enough to confirm that measles vaccine is a poor protector of infants' and children's health.

Table 11-1

14 INVESTIGATED OUTBREAKS OF MEASLES IN 1977

CASES IN VACCINATED*	PERCENT VACCINATED	CASES IN UNVACCINATED**	PERCENT UNVACCINATED
511	40.9%	737	59.1%

*history of previous measles vaccination
**no prior history of measles or measles vaccination

Source: Immunization Division, Bureau of State Services, and Field Services Division, Bureau of Epidemiology, Centers for Disease Control. *MMWR* 1977;26(14):109.

The medical evidence supports the view that the measles vaccine can actually make children more susceptible to wild measles virus caught naturally through contagion, because the vaccine antigen somehow desensitizes or weakens the child's immune response—especially if the same antigen is introduced into the body a second or third time. Measles vaccine, in many cases, simply does not provide immunity against future bouts of measles. What happens instead is that the vaccine interferes with the child's ability to gain a lasting protection or the type of immunity unvaccinated children achieve from contracting measles naturally. In my mind, the vaccinated are more susceptible to the adverse effects of measles should they catch the disease after being vaccinated. It seems to matter little whether vaccinated children become sick with measles, six days, six months, or six years after their immunization, because they were never properly protected in the first place. Since millions of children have been vaccinated for measles every year since 1963, it follows that all age groups of vaccinated individuals up to about age thirty-five are still susceptible. Moreover, expert medical evidence bears this out. Physicians began to report cases of atypical measles in 1965. In the 1970s, cases of atypical measles were occurring on average between ten and twelve years after vaccination with killed measles vaccine.[73] In one remarkable account of four siblings, who were all vaccinated with killed measles vaccines in 1963 and 1964 when they were between one and four years old, and whose medical history was monitored by physicians for many years, two of the four children were known to develop atypical measles in 1978 and 1979, sixteen years after receiving the killed measles vaccine. Moreover, the same two children had also received two doses of live measles vaccine in 1970 and 1974.[74] Thus, neither the primary measles vaccine series given in 1963 (3 doses: 2 killed, 1 attenuated), nor the two doses of live measles vaccine given in 1970 and 1974 respectively (5 doses total) failed to protect these children from the disease. Additionally, there are also reports from physicians that children who developed atypical measles were given a different diagnosis for the condition. These diagnoses included: Rocky Mountain spotted fever, rubella, viral pneumonia, acute appendicitis and other syndromes.[75] Meanwhile, unless the medical history of the child is really scrutinized, the connection between the vaccine and the disease is lost—or, in many cases, denied.

There are many unanswered questions about mass vaccination programs. I'm sure you're probably asking yourself, What about the millions of children who received measles vaccines and who never contracted measles afterwards? Doesn't that prove that the vaccine works and is protecting them from disease? Again, was it the vaccine that protected them or was it their own natural immunity and quality of health? Since the vaccine has demonstrated such a high failure rate, how could it possibly be successful at protecting millions from disease?

The reported number of cases of natural measles declined from about 400,000 a year in the early 1960s (before the vaccine) to about 30,000 a year by 1975 (after the vaccine), yet the measles death rate remained the same.[76] Although the measles vaccine (like all vaccines) has been given the credit for greatly reducing the incidence of disease, especially after mass vaccination programs began on a large scale, I question whether the vaccine could achieve this distinction in light of its fumbling track record. By way of comparison, the reported number of cases of chickenpox, another mild disease of childhood for which there is no vaccine, are about 150,000 to 200,000 each year.[77] However, this number represents only about 5 to 7 percent of actual cases.[78] It is estimated that about 3 million children in the United States have chickenpox each year.[79]

Chickenpox, like measles in the prevaccine era, has its highest attack rate in the five to nine age group and peaks in winter and spring.[80] One attack of chickenpox (like natural measles) provides life-long immunity; second attacks are rare.[81] Immunity following inapparent infections of chickenpox (without observable symptoms) is as good as immunity after the full-blown disease.[82] There are about one hundred chickenpox "associated" deaths in the United States each year from among 3,000,000 actual cases (33 deaths per million cases).

Judging from the historical characteristics of chickenpox, I suspect that the reported number of cases of measles today represents significant underreporting, just as was probably the situation in the 1950s. More importantly, if the measles vaccine were abandoned tomorrow, I believe the number of cases of natural measles (like those of chickenpox today) would sky-rocket. This strongly suggests that measles vaccine (like all vaccines) is not eradicating disease per se, but merely altering or suppressing it. Thus, the popularly held notion that vaccines can wipe out a disease or are presently eliminating the disease without presenting major complications in their wake, is highly unlikely. Along with great underreporting of disease generally, and the failure to report milder "modified" cases of measles in vaccinated children is the likelihood that measles vaccine may be simply aborting natural measles infections, altering and delaying their natural expression. While the vaccine gets the credit for eliminating the disease, it has only reshuffled it, recreated it, into something far more costly and debilitating—disease in later life.

CHAPTER 12

The Myth of
Vaccine Immunity

*T*he rationale that has been used by medical science to
validate the theory of immunization is based on the presence of antibodies. When a person is immunized for measles,
for example, the antibody that is produced in response to the
measles vaccine antigen can be detected and measured from
that person's blood sample. The level of measurable antibody
in the blood is called the antibody titre. Through sophisticated
testing, the antibody titre is detectable in blood serum six days,
six weeks, or even six years following a primary immunization
or booster shot. The presence of circulating antibody, even
years later, is one of the indicators that is used by medical
science to prove that infection with vaccine virus has indeed
taken place, and that immunity, or protection against disease,
is still active. It is this second point—that vaccine immunity is
still active or effective—that I have found to be false.

In 1913, Bela Schick, a Hungarian-born pediatrician and
bacteriologist, developed a test that allegedly determined whether
a person was susceptible or immune to diphtheria. During the
Schick test, a small amount of diphtheria toxin was injected
under the skin. If a red spot developed at the injection site,
indicating a positive reaction, the person was susceptible to
diphtheria. If the red spot failed to appear on the skin,
indicating a negative response, the person was immune to
diphtheria.

Leon Chaitow, one of Europe's leading naturopathic physicians and the author of *Vaccination and Immunization:*

Dangers, Delusions and Alternatives, points out that sufficient antitoxin in the blood following diphtheria immunization
does not necessarily mean that the person is immune to diphtheria.[1] In England, during the 1940s, diphtheria occurred in many
people who were inoculated with the vaccine. The Medical
Research Council of Great Britain led one investigative study in
which 40 percent of those vaccinated against diphtheria who
later contracted the disease had antitoxin concentrations greater
than Schick's standard dividing line.[2] Although they thus should
have been immune, they weren't. Conversely, others who were
not inoculated for diphtheria and showed no antitoxin in their
blood, escaped the disease. Similarly, people who were inoculated with diphtheria vaccine and demonstrated lower than
Schick's acceptable levels of antitoxin (including nurses working
on hospital diphtheria wards) also remained well. According to
the theory, both groups should have contracted the disease.

One of the alleged benefits of mass immunizations is that, in
addition to protecting large numbers of immunized children
from clinical disease, it protects the rest through "herd immunity." According to this theory, if a sizeable portion of a given
population (usually 75 percent or greater) is vaccinated against
a particular disease, this will protect the remaining susceptibles
in the population from contracting the disease by successfully
halting its spread. In 1964, when many adult women contracted
rubella (German measles) during their pregnancies and gave
birth in many cases to children with birth defects, a big push for
the licensure of a rubella vaccine took place. This was a
somewhat strange event, because rubella was—and has been—
a mild, non-fatal illness of childhood with very few complications.
Nevertheless, rubella vaccine was licensed in the United States
in 1969, and by the early 1970s mass rubella vaccination
programs were already under way. Because a percentage of
women of childbearing age were susceptible to rubella infection,
it was believed that by immunizing a large percentage of
children, perhaps 75 percent or more, herd immunity among
children would protect the 15 percent or so of adult childbearing

females who were susceptible to rubella infection. However, a number of studies that followed in the wake of mass rubella vaccination programs proved those "beliefs" to be false. One study demonstrated that in a given population, with 80 to 95 percent of the people immune to rubella, the remaining susceptibles were not prevented from contracting the disease.[3] In addition, the percentage of people who were vaccinated with rubella vaccine but reinfected a second time fluctuated, sometimes reaching as high as 80 percent.[4] However, less than 10 percent of those who contract rubella naturally (the nonvaccinated) suffer rubella a second time.[5] What is perplexing to many vaccine researchers is that strong levels of rubella antibodies have been detected in the blood of vaccinees for up to seven years following rubella vaccination, and yet a high number of vaccinated individuals become infected again, perhaps a number of times afterwards. Vincent Fulginiti, M.D., asks the crucial question: "How then does reinfection occur, if serum antibody is indicative of immunity!"[6] It seems apparent to me, although few will admit it, that the presence of serum antibody does not indicate foolproof protection against infection, reinfection, or disease, nor does it denote immunity. Neither does the lack of antibody mean, in all cases, that the individual will necessarily suffer the disease. Therefore, based on the evidence, the theory of vaccine protection, validated by the presence of antibody, is false. Moreover, it appears that herd immunity does not work.

The required amount of diphtheria antitoxin in the blood of vaccinated individuals still did not prevent clinical diphtheria from occurring, nor did the absence of it denote that the individuals were doomed to contract diphtheria; their own natural immunity protected them. Likewise, the presence of strong antibody to rubella virus in the blood of those vaccinated against rubella did not protect those individuals from reinfection with the wild rubella virus when they were reexposed. In both cases, the presence of antibody in the blood, the barometer by which vaccine immunity is measured, proved to be a false measure. The presence of antibody can no longer be used as proof of vaccine immunity. The scientific principle behind immunization does not stand up under scrutiny. In truth, immunization provides "artificial" immunity. It is temporary. It is fleeting. In fact, it may not exist at all.

CHAPTER 13

Vaccination and the Law

A lthough there is no blanket federal immunization law in the United States, the individual state statutes are remarkably uniform in content and application. What makes the immunization statutes so singularly alike is that they set mandatory conditions for school attendance. Compulsory immunization statutes require that all school-age children (except children with exemptions) be immunized before they can legally attend school. In general, this requirement applies to children entering school at the kindergarten level. However, since the advent of licensed day care, many states require children to be immunized at the preschool level.

A Historical Sketch

Edward Jenner, a country doctor from Gloucestershire, England, is credited with discovering vaccination in 1796. The practice was introduced in Massachusetts in 1800 by Benjamin Waterhouse, Professor of Physic (medicine) at Harvard College. In 1809 the Commonwealth of Massachusetts encouraged its towns to make provision for the inoculation of its inhabitants with cow pox vaccine and empowered the boards of health to raise money to defray the costs.[1] By 1855, the compulsory nature of the vaccination statute was already firm. Here are some excerpts from the Massachusetts statute of 1855:

SECT. I.   Parents and guardians of youth, shall cause the children under their care to be vaccinated before they attain the age of two years.

SECT. II.   The school committee of the several towns and cities, shall not allow any child to be admitted to, or connected with the public schools, who has not been duly vaccinated.

SECT. III.   The selectmen of the several towns, and the mayor and aldermen of every city, shall enforce the vaccination of all the inhabitants of said town and cities, and every parent or guardian of youth who shall not cause his or her child or ward to be vaccinated, (the said child or ward being more than two years of age,) shall be liable to a fine of five dollars for each and every year's neglect, to be recovered on complaint of the selectmen of the town, or of the mayor and aldermen of the city, for the benefit and use of said town or city.[2]

The compulsory aspect of vaccination has had a long-standing history in the United States and in Europe. In the United States vaccination statutes were originally created as a public health measure to protect infants and children from smallpox. Because many in the medical profession strongly believed that vaccination was the best method of preventing smallpox and reducing communicable disease, the belief became common and was adopted by state legislatures and translated into law at the turn of the twentieth century. Even though there was strong opposition to smallpox vaccination among some physicians, clergyman, and untold thousands of common citizens, they could not compete with the influential current of medical opinion at that time. By 1905, however, only eleven states had compulsory vaccination statutes, while thirty-four did not.[3] Moreover, none of the states physically forced vaccination on their citizens; three-quarters of the states did not enforce legal penalties, and Utah and West Virginia expressed the view that no force or compulsion be used on their citizens.[4]

What is singularly astounding about smallpox vaccination is that it was made compulsory apparently without state legislatures properly scrutinizing its history.[5] The same could be said of the situation in Western Europe, where smallpox vaccination was compulsory and rigorously practiced, and smallpox deaths plentiful during the second half of the nineteenth century.

In England, vaccination was made compulsory in 1853 and enforceable by fine in 1867.[6] In Birmingham, one of the most vaccinated cities in England, the preventive power of smallpox vaccine was apparently nonexistent. Dr. Alfred Hill, medical officer of health, reports that for the period 1871 to 1874 there were 7,706 cases of smallpox in Birmingham; of these, 6,795 had been vaccinated.[7] In 1871, in Bavaria, Germany, where vaccination was compulsory and revaccination commonplace, there were 30,472 cases of smallpox; of these, 29,429 were vaccinated.[8]

A brief glance at England in the period from 1854 to 1874 reveals that there was optimum public vaccination coverage imposed by compulsory law, estimated to be 75 percent of live births during the years 1853 to 1860.[9] Vaccination reached more than 90 percent of the population in many poor working-class parishes of London, especially after 1867 when non-payment of vaccination fines resulted in harsh penalties. Nonetheless, smallpox deaths increased significantly throughout the period, and England suffered three of the worst smallpox epidemics of the nineteenth century: 1857 to 1859, 1863 to 1865, and 1870 to 1872.

Table 13-1

DEATHS FROM SMALLPOX IN ENGLAND AND WALES

Date of Epidemic	Deaths from Smallpox
1857-1859	14,244
1863-1865	20,059
1870-1872	44,840

Increase of population from 1st to 2nd epidemic, **7** percent.
Increase of smallpox in the same period, nearly **50** percent.
Increase of population from 2nd to 3rd epidemic, **10** percent.
Increase of smallpox in the same period, **120** percent.

Table 13-1 continued

DEATHS FROM SMALLPOX (BY DECADE) IN ENGLAND AND WALES FOLLOWING COMPULSORY VACCINATION REQUIREMENTS

1854-1863 33,515
1864-1873 70,458

Source: C.T. Pearce, M.D. Vital Statistics, no. 1, February 1877, cited in W. Young and G. Wilkinson, *Vaccination Tracts: Facts and Figures* (Providence: Snow and Farnham, 1892), p.3.

Police Powers

Compulsory vaccination statutes were created to protect the public from the spread of communicable disease.[10] The enforcement of vaccination statutes falls within the legal boundaries of a state's police powers, or the inherent authority of a governing body to impose reasonable restrictions on its citizens for the general benefit, welfare, and safety of all. During the last eighty-five years there have been many attempts to challenge the validity of compulsory vaccination statutes. The case that is most often cited as authority in the matter is *Jacobson v. Massachusetts*.

Jacobson v. Massachusetts

In 1902, because smallpox was prevalent in the city of Cambridge, Massachusetts, the Board of Health passed an ordinance requiring all inhabitants of Cambridge to be vaccinated for smallpox. Those citizens who were already vaccinated were exempt—provided that they had received the vaccine during the last five years. Others who had received the vaccine earlier were subject to revaccination.[11]

Henning Jacobson, an adult citizen of Cambridge, had been vaccinated for smallpox in his childhood and had suffered a serious and prolonged reaction to the vaccine.[12] Years later, his son also suffered an adverse reaction. When the city ordinance was passed, Jacobson not only refused to be revaccinated for smallpox, but refused to pay the $5 fine for non-compliance. His case went before a trial court and was later appealed to the Supreme Judicial Court of Massachusetts. The trial court returned a verdict of guilty and the appellate court affirmed the jury verdict. In 1904 *Jacobson v. Massachusetts* went before the United States Supreme Court, the only vaccination case to date to reach the highest court.

During his U. S. Supreme Court trial, Jacobson argued that the Massachusetts vaccination statute was in violation of his personal liberties secured by the Fourteenth Amendment of the U.S. Constitution, in particular, the clause: "No state shall make or enforce any law abridging the privileges or immunities of citizens of the United States; nor shall any state deprive any person of life, liberty or property without due process of law, nor deny to any person within its jurisdiction the equal protection of the laws."[13] He also argued that to fine or imprison someone for refusing to be vaccinated admits to the unreasonableness and oppressive nature of the compulsory vaccination statute and is an assault upon his person. In further comments, he focused on the unreliability of smallpox vaccine to prevent smallpox in all cases, and the inherent dangers the vaccine presented to a person's health; he used his son and himself as examples. His attorney argued that even if Jacobson had presented expert medical testimony from a physician [which he did not], who could show that smallpox vaccination would be detrimental to his health, the "law recognized no such defense" and so it must be excluded as evidence.[14] His attorney also asserted that the Massachusetts vaccination statute violated equal protection of the law. During that time, in Massachusetts, physicians were permitted to exempt children from smallpox vaccine if the physician felt the vaccine would be injurious to the child's health. Adults did not enjoy that same exemption.[15] Finally, Jacobson's attorney argued that to be forced by law to introduce disease (vaccine) into a healthy body was not only a violation of liberty, but if the person were injured as a result, it constituted damage without compensation.[16]

While the arguments presented by Jacobson and counsel were strong ones, they could not overcome the power invested in a state or governing body (police power) to enforce laws necessary for the general health and welfare of its citizens. The Supreme Court took the position that the individual liberties of a single person are not absolute and must give way to reasonable restraint, in certain circumstances, when the safety, comfort and welfare of the majority are of issue, or "not permit the interests of the many to be subordinated to the wishes or convenience of the few."[17]

Smallpox Prevention

The issue of whether smallpox vaccination was the best method of preventing smallpox was not the immediate point of debate. The Supreme Court addressed the issue, nonetheless, by defining the scope of a "common belief":

> It must be conceded," it said," that some layman, both learned and unlearned, and some physicians of great skill and repute, do not believe that vaccination is a preventive of smallpox. . . . While not accepted by all, it is accepted by the mass of people, as well as by most members of the medical profession. . . . While we do not decide and cannot decide that vaccination is a preventative of smallpox, we take judicial notice of the fact that this is the common belief of the people of the State, and with this fact as a foundation we hold that the statute in question is a health law, enacted as a reasonable and proper exercise of police power.[18]

During its closing remarks, in somewhat of a twist, the Supreme Court remarked that it did not hold "absolute" that an adult must be vaccinated for smallpox if the individual could demonstrate that he was an unfit subject for vaccination at the time of his vaccination and that his unfit condition would "seriously impair his health or probably cause his death."[19] Although Henning Jacobson and his son both suffered severely from smallpox vaccinations, apparently, because Jacobson was presently in "perfect" health, the court made its final remark, "no such case is seen here."[20]

Jacobson v. Massachusetts has had a major impact on subsequent cases that have challenged the constitutionality of compulsory vaccination statutes. Moreover, the weighty decision in *Jacobson* has been used successfully to overcome arguments that have tried to establish that compulsory vaccination statutes violate a child's right to attend public school.[21] In *Freeman v. Zimmerman* the courts maintained that compulsory vaccination statutes, which deal with the health and safety of its citizens, take precedence, and that compulsory education statutes are subordinate to vaccination statutes.[22] While arguments against compulsory immunization based on the First Amendment right of freedom of religion have afforded parents and their children relief from school immunization requirements in the form of a religious exemption, less than 2 percent of the population take advantage of this legal waiver (see chapter 14, table 14-1). In any event, the case of *Jacobson v. Massachusetts* has been used repeatedly, with much success, to defend the actions of states to exercise police powers especially when the constitutionality of compulsory vaccination statutes were at stake.

CHAPTER 14

How To Legally Avoid
Immunization

S chool children in the United States are required to be
immunized before they can attend school. Yet this requirement is not without exceptions. The *State Immunization
Requirements for School Children,* published in 1981 by the
United States Public Health Service, notes that state statutes
allow parents and guardians and their children three categories
of exemptions from childhood immunizations: (1) medical, (2)
religious, and (3) philosophical.[1]

THE MEDICAL EXEMPTION

In the United States, medical exemptions are defined by the
statements and opinions of physicians.[2] Those authorized
include medical doctors (M.D.'s) and doctors of osteopathy
(D.O.'s). If a physician determines that an immunization may be
detrimental to a child's health and expresses that opinion in
writing, a medical exemption is created. Although health
departments have the power to veto a medical exemption, and
do so on occasion, they usually do not question the physicians's
authority.

Some medical exemptions are temporary, while others are
permanent. This determination is based on the status of a
child's health at the time of immunization. Children may have
an immunization shot delayed, because of a prevailing health
condition, only to receive the vaccine a year or two later. Other
children, for example, may receive MMR vaccine but not DPT.
In theory, children in fragile health are exempt from all shots.

School immunization requirements are uniform among most states and require that temporary medical exemptions be reevaluated every year or so. Children and their parents must comply with state immunization statutes and school superintendents must comply with health department regulations that demand an accurate accounting in the schools of who is and who is not immunized.

Medical exemptions were written into state compulsory vaccination statutes in the nineteenth century to protect children in fragile health from the possible serious adverse effects of the smallpox vaccine. Because the effect of a vaccine on any infant is in part unpredictable, however, there is no way to determine who is going to react adversely to it. The medical profession uses a few general guidelines which loosely determine who should not be vaccinated.

Physicians and drug manufacturers use the word "contraindicated" to describe medical situations or conditions under which vaccines should be delayed or not used at all. In general, a vaccine is contraindicated when the child's immune system is suppressed as a result of serious illness such as: active tuberculosis, leukemia, lymphomas, or malignant neoplasms (abnormal growth-tumor) that affect the bone or lymphatic system. A vaccine can also be contraindicated if the infant or child is taking certain medications that lower resistance to infection; among these medications are cortisone, prednisone, and certain anti-cancer drugs. A vaccine is also contraindicated in an individual who has had a prior serious reaction. Other grounds for medical exemption are allergies to substances in the vaccine. The most common substances in vaccines to which infants and children could be allergic are: egg protein, thimerosal (mercury-preservative), aluminum sulfate (adjuvant), and neomycin-streptomycin (antibiotics used in trace amounts).

Each vaccine has its own individual precautions. The following is a list of contraindications for the DPT, rubella, MMR, OPV, and hemophilus influenzae vaccines. It represents a cross section of data from the Immunization Practices Advisory

Committee (ACIP), vaccine manufacturers, and the United States Public Health Service.[3]

VACCINE CONTRAINDICATIONS

DPT (diphtheria-pertussis-tetanus)

1. Sickness at the time of scheduled vaccinations with something more serious than a cold
2. History of convulsions or suspicion of nervous system problems
3. Serious prior reaction to DPT, DT, or TD shots, such as an allergic reaction to any vaccine component; a temperature of 105° F or greater following the shots; an episode of limpness and paleness; prolonged continuous crying; an unusual, high-pitched cry; or a convulsion or other more severe problem of the brain
4. Use of a drug or participation in treatment that lowers the body's resistance to infection, such as cortisone, prednisone, certain anti-cancer drugs, or irradiation
5. An immediate anaphylactic reaction (hypersensitivity to a foreign substance)
6. Collapse or shock-like state within forty-eight hours of receiving the vaccine
7. Encephalopathy (not due to another identifiable cause), defined as an acute, severe central nervous system disorder occurring within seven days after vaccination and generally consisting of major alterations in consciousness, unreponsiveness, or generalized or focal seizures that persist more than a few hours, without recovery within twenty-four hours.

Rubella (german measles)

1. Pregnancy or plans for pregnancy within three months of having received the vaccine
2. Current respiratory illness or "active febrile infection"
3. Treatment with immunosuppressive therapy or presence of the following health disorders:
   a. Blood dyscrasia (toxic materials in the blood)
   b. Leukemia
   c. Lymphomas (any type)
   d. Active untreated tuberculosis
   e. Malignant neoplasms (growths-tumors) affecting the bone marrow or lymphatic system

MMR (measles-mumps-rubella)

1. Hypersensitivity to eggs, with reactions such as hives, difficult breathing, hypotension, throat swellings, and shock
2. Known hypersensitivity to neomycin (antibiotic)
3. Pregnancy or plans for pregnancy within three months of vaccination.
4. "Family history of congenital or hereditary immunodeficiency, until the immune competence of the vaccine recipient is demonstrated"
5. Active febrile infection or respiratory illness or lymphomas of any kind

OPV (oral polio vaccine)

1. Acute illness or "advance condition," or persistent vomiting or diarrhea
2. Immune deficiency or altered immune states such as leukemia, lymphoma, or thymic abnormalities (Avoidance after receiving OPV, of contact with household members with altered immune systems, is also recommended.)

3. Lowered resistance caused by therapy with corticosteriods, alkalating drugs, radiation, or antimetabolites
4. Immunodeficiency within the family
5. Pregnancy

Haemophilus Influenzae

1. Sensitivity to the materials in the vaccine, including thimerosal (preservative) and diphtheria toxoid
2. Presence of any illness accompanied by fever or acute infection
3. Contraindication in the event of pregnancy is unclear

The problem with medical exemptions is that they cover too narrow a range of symptoms. It is not difficult to figure out that an infant who has had a convulsion (in many cases from previous DPT inoculations) should not receive more DPT, when the vaccine is known to produce convulsive seizures. It has been noted in many vaccine publications of the Centers For Disease Control that a vaccine is contraindicated for "anyone who is sick at the time of vaccination with anything more serious than a cold."[4] But what about an infant with a cold? The immune system is unquestionably compromised during a cold. Are some infants given vaccine when they have a cold or are recovering from one? One also wonders about all the children with asthma? Should they be immunized? According to current vaccine recommendations, they are candidates to receive vaccine inoculations. None of these children should be getting a vaccine.

The medical guidelines for determining whether a child should receive an immunization shot are too arbitrary, because they screen out only high-risk children. The truth is that perfectly healthy babies suffer severe reactions from vaccines. There is no way of knowing if your child is going to be one of these children. In the United States, fewer than 1 percent of infants and children are granted medical exemptions from immunizations.[5] However, a number of vaccinated babies suffer severe, life-crippling reactions each year. In 1984, Assistant Secretary of Health Edward Brandt Jr., M.D., testified before the U.S. Senate Committee on Labor and Human Resources that there were 9,000 cases of convulsions, 9,000 cases of collapse and 17,000 cases of high-pitched screaming episodes— or a total of 35,000 cases of acute neurological reactions occurring in American infants and children each year within forty-eight hours of a DPT vaccine.[6] If about 3.3 million children were vaccinated for DPT in 1984 and 35,000 infants and children suffered neurological reactions from the vaccine, this represents 1 percent of healthy babies suffering severe reactions to a vaccine for which a medical exemption was not forthcoming. It has been ascertained by a number of reliable studies that perhaps 1/3 of the 35,000 children (or 11,666 children) will have lingering long-term conditions as a result of the DPT vaccine, including uncontrollable seizure disorders, mental retardation, learning disabilities, hyperactivity, behavior problems, and chronic systemic illness.[7] Of the 3.3 million newborns vaccinated for DPT each year in the U.S., about 943 will be killed by the vaccine, although a second estimate puts the total at slightly over 2,000.[8] As staggering as these numbers are, they don't include the more than 1 1/2 million infants each year who have local or systemic reactions to the DPT vaccine. Such reactions are estimated to occur in between 50 and 64 percent of all vaccinated babies. (UCLA-FDA study) These adverse reactions are viewed by the medical profession as acceptable and are not counted in the tallies when benefits versus risks are evaluated.

Thus, because the medical contraindications cover too narrow a range of conditions and do not address the problem of severe reactions suffered by healthy babies, the medical exemption is an imperfect measure for screening susceptible children from vaccine injury.

THE RELIGIOUS EXEMPTION

The religious exemption offers parents the most accessible way to legally avoid immunizations for their children. The religious exemption clause is written into childhood immunization statutes in every state, with the exception of West Virginia and Mississippi.

The Religious Exemption in Massachusetts

In Massachusetts, where I live, the religious exemption was added to the General Laws as a statutory amendment in 1967 and was largely the effort of the Church of Christ, Scientist, to legally exempt its church members from immunization requirements.[9] Since Christian Scientists eschew the use of drugs or serums and believe in the power of prayer as a means of spiritual healing, it was fitting that they finally secured a religious exemption.

The religious exemption in Massachusetts has not been without its problems, however. The main point of dispute was the statutory wording that excluded people with sincere religious beliefs who were not members or adherents of an organized church or religious denomination. The religious exemption clause (1967) in Massachusetts read:

> In the absence of an emergency or epidemic of disease declared by the department of public health, no child whose parent or guardian objects in writing to vaccination or immunization upon the ground that it conflicts with the tenets and practice of a recognized church or religious denomination of which he is an adherent or member shall be required to present said physician's certificate in order to be admitted to school, but may present, in lieu thereof, an affidavit signed by an official of such church or religious denomination that the parent or guardian of such child is an adherent or member in good standing of such church or religious denomination

and that such parent or guardian objects on religious grounds to vaccination and immunization.[10]

Dalli v. Board of Education

In 1969, Beula Dalli, who was not a member of any church, brought suit against the Board of Education claiming that the current religious exemption statute in Massachusetts prevented her from obtaining a religious exemption for her daughter because it would be impossible to get the necessary signature from a church official. She charged that the statute deprived her and her daughter of equal protection of the law and the free exercise of religion.[11] Ms. Dalli, whose personal beliefs were based "in the Bible and its teachings" was opposed to vaccination "as a matter of conscience."[12] She was also opposed to the "injection of animal serum" because this violated her Bible lessons' warnings to "keep the body clean and acceptable to God."[13] The Massachusetts Supreme Judicial Court ruled that the third paragraph of the immunization statute extended preferential treatment to members or adherents of a "recognized church" but denied it to all others whose objections to vaccination were also "grounded in religious belief."[14] The Court found that this preferential treatment of one group over the other violated the First and Fourteenth Amendment of the United States Constitution and Article 2 of the Declaration of Rights of the Massachusetts Constitution.[15] Therefore the third paragraph having to do with "members or adherents of a recognized church" was declared unconstitutional and was stricken from the statute. Since 1971, the new wording of the religious exemption clause has been:

> In the absence of an emergency or epidemic of disease declared by the Department of Public Health no child whose parent or guardian states in writing that vaccination or immunization conflicts with his sincere religious beliefs shall be required to present said physician's certificate in order to be admitted to school.[16]

The decision rendered in *Dalli* v. *Board of Education* demonstrated that an individual's sincere religious beliefs were valid in opposing immunizations. The court said: "It is not our function to pass on the merits of the plaintiff's beliefs. No matter how misguided or even ridiculous such beliefs may appear to be to the court, or to the overwhelming majority of people, unless they damage a compelling state interest the courts can examine only to determine if they are sincerely held."[17]

Dalli v. *Board of Education* strengthened and clarified the broader meaning of a religious belief embodied in the First Amendment. More importantly, it allowed parents in Massachusetts who held sincere religious beliefs the legal right to oppose immunization in a simple and straightforward manner, whether they belonged to a church or not.

The Religious Exemption In New York

In the state of New York, where the religious exemption has been on the books since 1966, the exemption, as in Massachusetts, was available only to "bona fide members of a recognized religious organization," but not to others with sincere religious beliefs.[18] During the last decade a number of individuals whose religious exemption was denied by local school districts in New York challenged the exemption statute in court. Some have been successful, while others have not.

In *Sherr* v. *Northport-East Northport Union Free School District*, two families, the Sherrs and the Levys, sought relief from the immunization of their children under New York's Public Health Law, Section 2164(9), the religious exemption statute.[19] The court granted the Levys a religious exemption for their daughter but refused the Sherr family one for their son.

In the *Sherr* case, the court asserted that Alan Sherr's beliefs against vaccination were derived from his "medical and philosophical perspective as a chiropractor and chiropractic ethics not from any religiously inspired source."[20] Sherr joined a church in Florida called the Missionary Temple at Large, Universal Religious Brotherhood, Inc., which was opposed to immunizations. However, further investigation revealed that the temple was run out of the minister's house, held no religious services, had no formal organizational structure, and in the words of the court was a "mail order church."[21] The Sherrs' request for a religious exemption was denied.[22]

The Levy family, on the other hand, demonstrated that they had studied religion and spirituality for many years and that they embraced those religious principles in their daily lives. More importantly, the Levys exemplified a sincerity about their religious convictions and way of life that impressed the court. The Levys, like the Sherrs, joined a church, in their case the Church of Human Life Science, in order to facilitate the exemption. The court maintained that this church was not a "sham" and that the Levy's beliefs were in line with the church's religious teachings such as "the integrity of the body be maintained" since "our bodies are the temple of our being" and that "all drugs and vaccines are ethically, morally, religiously, mentally and physically wrong, being at variance with our Creator's Mandate."[23] As a result, the court ruled that the previous denial of the Levys' religious exemption by the school district violated the family's constitutional rights and held that the Levys were entitled to a religious exemption.[24] Furthermore, the court ruled that the clause in New York Public Health Law 2164(9) "bona fide members of a recognized religious organization" was "blatantly unconstitutional."[25] In the future the statute must "offer the exemption to all persons who sincerely hold religious beliefs that prohibit the inoculation of their children by the state."[26]

In yet another vaccination case, *Mason v. General Brown Central School District* the plaintiffs, Dr. Edgar Mason, a chiropractor, and his spouse, Karen Mason of Watertown, New York, were denied the religious exemption they sought for their son.[27] Although the Masons had joined a chartered branch of the Universal Life Church whose teachings were opposed to immunizations, the court found it questionable that the church had no membership requirements, no traditional doctrine, or regular worship services. Anyone could become an "ecclesiastical leader" in the church by simply paying a five dollar fee.[28]

Second, the court maintained that the Masons' beliefs, which were based on a "genetic blueprint," were primarily scientific rather than religious, and so their religious exemption was denied them.

Thus, in New York, where some parents' religious exemption letters have been scrutinized by school districts and later litigated in court, there appears to be no set formula for determining a religious exemption; each case stands on its own merit. It appears from these cases that one must have religious beliefs that are sincerely held and occupy a dominant place in the individual's life.

How to Claim a Religious Exemption

The requirement for filing a religious exemption is simple and straightforward. The majority of states asks that you (on behalf of your child) write a statement or short letter to the school principal (in some states to the health department) declaring that immunization conflicts with your sincere religious principles or beliefs. You do not have to go into detail about your religious beliefs to fulfill this requirement. A simple declaration against immunizations is all that is required (in most cases) to gain the religious exemption. You should also include in your letter:

1. Your child's name
2. A statement that you as parent or legal guardian assume full responsibility for the health of your child
3. The date
4. Your signature

In addition, some states require that the exemption letter be notarized. (It wouldn't hurt to have all exemption-related letters you write notarized.)

Here is a sampling of the religious exemption statutes for ten states including: Arkansas, Colorado, Florida, Indiana, Massachusetts, Michigan, New Hampshire, Ohio, Texas, and

Wisconsin. These states were picked at random and cover many geographical areas of the United States.

Arkansas

The provisions of this section shall not apply if the parents or legal guardian of that child object thereto on the grounds that such immunization conflicts with the religious tenets and practices of a recognized church or religious denomination of which the parent or guardian is an adherent or member. Furthermore, the provisions of this section requiring pertussis vaccination shall not apply to any child with a sibling, either whole blood or half blood, who has had a serious adverse reaction to the pertussis antigen which reaction resulted in a total permanent disability.[29]

Colorado

Upon submitting a statement signed by one parent or guardian or the emancipated child that the parent, guardian, or child is an adherent to a religious belief whose teachings are opposed to immunizations or that the parent or guardian or the emancipated child has a personal belief that is opposed to immunizations.[30]

Florida

The parent or guardian of the child objects in writing that the administration of immunizing agents conflicts with his religious tenets or practices.[31]

Indiana

Except as otherwise provided, no school child shall be required to undergo any testing, examination, immunization or treatment required under this chapter when his parent objects. An objection will not exempt a child from any testing, examination, immunization or treatment required under this chapter unless it is made in writing, signed by the child's parent and delivered to the child's teacher or to the individual who might order a test, exam, immunization or treatment absent the objection.[32]

Massachusetts

In the absence of an emergency or epidemic of disease declared by the Department of Public Health, no child whose parent or guardian states in writing that vaccination or immunization conflicts with his sincere religious beliefs shall be required to present said physician's certificate in order to be admitted to school.[33]

Michigan

A child is exempt from this part if a parent, guardian, or person in loco parentis of the child presents a written statement to the administrator of the child's school or operator of the group program to the effect that the requirements of this part cannot be met because of religious convictions or other objection to immunization.[34]

New Hampshire

A child shall be exempt from immunization if a parent or legal guardian objects to immunization because of religious beliefs. The parent or legal guardian shall sign a notarized form stating that the child has not been immunized because of religious beliefs.[35]

Ohio

A pupil who presents a written statement of his parent or guardian in which the parent or guardian objects to the immunization for good cause, including religious convictions, is not required to be immunized.[36]

Texas

The child or student must present an affidavit signed by the applicant, or if a minor, by his or her parent or guardian stating that the immunization conflicts with the tenets and practice of a recognized church or religious denomination of which the applicant is an adherent or member; provided, however, that this exemption does not apply in times of emergency or outbreak declared by the Commissioner of Health or local health authority.[37]

Wisconsin

The immunization requirement is waived if the student, if an adult, or the student's parent, guardian or legal custodian submits a written statement to the school, day care center or nursery school objecting to the immunization for reasons of health, religion or personal conviction. At the time any school, day care center or nursing school notifies a student, parent, guardian or legal custodian of the immunization requirements, it shall inform the person in writing of the person's right to a waiver under this paragraph.[38]

A number of other states do not ask for a religious exemption letter but prepare their own Certificate of Exemption form, as it is sometimes called. This is a "generalized" religious exemption statement that applies to all parents in that state who seek a religious exemption for their child. Sometimes this religious exemption statement is printed on the child's school health card or is part of the school immunization record card. In both cases, the parent or guardian simply signs the statement. Here is an example:

Parent or guardian of the above-named child adheres to a religious doctrine whose teachings are opposed to immunization.

Signed _____ Date _____
(Parent or guardian)

New Mexico and Vermont have combined the religious exemption with a philosophical exemption. In Vermont the exemption reads:

Religious or Moral Exemption
I request that immunization for my child be waived because they conflict with free exercise of religious or moral rights.[39]

_____
(Signature of parent or guardian)   (Telephone)   (D a t e)

Declare Your Opposition to Immunization in Writing

The most important element of declaring your opposition to immunization is that it MUST BE MADE IN WRITING to be valid. It is not enough that you telephone the school principal or personally inform the school nurse that you do not want immunization shots for your child.

The number of adults who exercise their legal right to seek a medical, religious, or philosophical exemption for their children in compliance with their state statutes is exceedingly small, less than 2 percent (see table 14-1). This may have some direct bearing on why the majority of religious exemption letters are accepted without argument or complications. However, I have heard of cases where a school principal or health department official challenged a letter or denied a religious exemption. This situation (as well as the need to go to court) can generally be avoided or remedied by doing a little planning and by cooperative work with school officials.

Why Some Religious Exemptions are Denied

When a religious exemption letter is challeged or denied by health authorities many times it is because it was not "properly worded." I strongly suggest that before drafting their exemption statement, parents write their state's health department requesting a copy of the school immunization statutes and explaining that they want to file for an exemption.   The departments usually send such information promptly.   The exemption statutes are short, easy to read, and well worth the small effort involved. By having them at your disposal you will be able to read the exact wording of the exemption and be able to frame your statement accordingly.

Since most large religious denominations in the U.S. have not openly taken a stand on immunization, a person who is a member of those churches (or a person who has no church affiliation whatsoever) would have to look elsewhere to qualify for a religious exemption in those states that make church membership a requirement for gaining a religious exemption. However, this should not deter anyone with sincere religious beliefs (in these states) from seeking an exemption. In order to qualify for the exemption, individuals need to be either members or "adherents" of a religious denomination whose teachings are opposed to immunization. Individuals might explore religions that are opposed to immunization to learn if their beliefs are compatible with yours. The decision to join a church is obviously a very personal one. However, one does not need to join the church to fulfill the religious exemption requirement. One need only to be an "adherent" of the church or religious denomination whose teachings are opposed to immunization.

Table 14-1

THE PERCENTAGE OF MEDICAL, RELIGIOUS AND PHILOSOPHICAL EXEMPTIONS TO VACCINATION, 25 U.S. STATES, 1989-1990

STATE	RELIGIOUS	MEDICAL	COMBINED REL./MED.	COMBINED REL./PHIL.
Arizona			.3%	
California		.1%		.5%
Colorado	.2%	.1%		1.1%
Florida	.3%	.5%		
Hawaii	.08%	.1%		
Illinois	.13%			
Indiana		.3%		.3%
Iowa	.25%	.27%		
Kentucky			.2%	
Maryland			1%	
Massachusetts			.5%	
Mississippi		.03%		
Missouri			3.3%	
Nevada	.2%	.9%		
New Hampshire	.3%	.2%		
New Jersey			.2%	
North Dakota	.16%	.07%		
Ohio			.2%	
Pennsylvania	.7%	.1%		
Tennessee			.1%	
Texas	.04%	.05%		
Utah			1.6%	
Vermont		.002%		.01%
Virginia	.2%	1%		
Washington	.2%	.2%		2.2%

2% = 2 exemptions for every 100 students.
.2% = 2 exemptions for every 1,000 students.
.02% = 2 exemptions for every 10,000 students.

Source: State Health Departments, July-August 1990. See also page 158.

Personal Religious Beliefs

As awareness grows that immunization can be opposed on the grounds that it conflicts with sincere religious beliefs, more people will probably explore the question of whether their own beliefs may, in fact, be "religious." In *Allanson v. Clinton School District*, Robert and Kathryn Allanson, neither of whom belonged to any church and who followed a macrobiotic philosophy and lifestyle, successfully secured a religious exemption for their children on the basis of their sincerely held personal religious beliefs.[40] Their suit helped bring into focus the expanded meaning of a personal religious belief embodied in the First Amendment. Although there is no "strict" definition of a personal religious belief, there are guidelines that help to define one.[41]

1. A person's religious belief may, but doesn't have to, include belief in a Deity
2. A person's religious belief must be chief in importance in a person's life
3. A person must be living by these beliefs

Consequently, a person's religious beliefs may encompass views on nature, spiritualism, and/or the scriptures and still be valid to oppose immunizations.[42] Most importantly, a person's religious beliefs or convictions must be sincerely held and hold a dominant place in the individual's life.

THE PHILOSOPHICAL EXEMPTION

Because there is a fine line between a personal religious belief and a belief that is essentially one of personal conscience, a number of states introduced the "philosophical" exemption to oppose immunization. Any individual who wishes to oppose immunization because it conflicts with personal beliefs, philosophy, conscience, or moral convictions may be granted relief from immunization by claiming a philosophical exemption against it. As of December 1992, twenty states offer a philosophical exemption. They are: Arizona, California,

Colorado, Idaho, Indiana, Louisiana, Maine, Michigan, Minnesota, Missouri, Nebraska, New Mexico, North Dakota, Ohio, Oklahoma, Rhode Island, Utah, Vermont, Washington, and Wisconsin.[43] The personal belief exemption is the easiest way to avoid unwanted immunizations. People who are opposed to immunizations and live in these twenty states should take full advantage of this opportunity.

What to do if Your Exemption is Denied

The greatest majority of requests for exemptions are honored. If your exemption is denied by school or health officials, ask them to give you their refusal in writing. Some school districts can be sticklers about the "wording" of exemption statements. In many cases the rearranging of certain key words or using different phrases has been the difference between success and failure. If the exemption is challenged, ask the school principal why it was denied. Let the principal know that you want to cooperate to successfully meet compliance with the immunization statute. Ask how you could best accomplish this. Often, by submitting a second, revised exemption statement, you will gain the exemption.

However, there are principals, school nurses, and other health administrators who believe that all children, bar none, must get vaccinated. They think nothing of harassing someone who doesn't agree with their rigidly held view. They will use scare tactics or try to make you feel guilty, implying that if you refuse vaccination, your child is going to get a serious disease. The issue here is your legal right to meet compliance with the vaccination statute by choosing an exemption, if you decide to do so. If however, your exemption is denied by the school principal, contact the school superintendent. If the superintendent does not give you any satisfaction I would contact your local school board. Ask that your request for a religious exemption be placed on the agenda. At some point you will present your case to the board and it will vote on your request. Make sure you get a decision in writing. If your request for a religious exemption is denied by the school board, I would suggest contacting an attorney. You have every right to object to immunizations if they violate your sincere religious beliefs. Be firm and don't let anyone sway you or disregard your inner feelings or convictions. Remember, the law is on your side. It's just that no one will tell you it is.

CHAPTER 15

The Protective Factors in Breast Milk

A side from love and care, there is no greater gift a mother can give her infant to protect against allergies, childhood infections, and disease than her breast milk. Breast milk contains vitamins, proteins, minerals, enzymes, hormones, and antibodies in the right proportion for the development, growth, and protection of the infant.

Research on the anti-infective properties of human breast milk is extensive and stretches from the 1930s to the present. Breast milk has proven to inhibit the growth of many bacteria and viruses in laboratory experiments. Antibodies or isoagglutinins have been isolated from breast milk in response to the following disease organisms: tetanus; pertussis; pneumonia; diphtheria; polio virus 1, 2, and 3; mumps; Coxsackie and echo virus; smallpox; and influenza organisms.[1]

Colostrum

The first milk that is secreted by mothers during the second half of pregnancy and for the first few days after giving birth is called colostrum. Colostrum is a lemon-yellowish milk that is very rich in protein and contains milk cells; vitamins A, E, B6, and B12; calcium; zinc; and immunoglobulins (antibodies).[2] Colostrum is so rich in protective nutrients that it is essential for a newborn to be given the opportunity to suck up as much colostrum milk as it desires during the first few hours and days following birth. As more colostrum is consumed by the baby, this satisfies one of the baby's strongest needs—to suck. The reflex action of the suckling infant stimulates the production of breast milk in the mother. The ingestion of colostrum also has a laxative effect and helps expel meconium, a greenish-black material found in the first stools discharged by newborns.[3]

The Antibodies in Breast Milk

The protective antibodies in colostrum and in later breast milk are derived from all classes of immunoglobulins, especially IgG, IgM, and IgA. The greatest concentration of antibody in breast milk is IgA.

The immunoglobulin IgA is referred to as secretory IgA (sIgA) and is somewhat different from the IgA that is produced in serum. The secretory immunoglobulin found in breast milk is thought to be produced in the mammary gland of the mother. SIgA greatly benefits breast-feeding infants because it coats their intestinal tract with an "antiseptic paint," thus protecting the infant from bacterial and viral invasions from such pathogens as E. coli, poliovirus, streptococci, staphylococci, and pneumococci.

The greatest concentration of secretory IgA is found in colostrum milk during the first day after delivery, and levels remain high for the next four or five days.[4] In 1978 S. Ogra, M.D. and P. Ogra, M.D., researchers in pediatrics and microbiology at Children's Hospital in Buffalo, New York, did extensive research on the antibody content of colostrum, mature breast milk, and serum of lactating mothers. They found significant levels of IgA, IgG, and IgM in the breast milk and the serum of the women for a full six months following birth.[5] Because the specific antiviral and antibacterial properties of colostrum milk were already well known, the authors suggested that breast-feeding during the first week after birth is crucial in providing the infant with "high concentrations of a wide variety of antibodies at time when the mucosal immune system has a poor level of function."[6]

Colostrum contains the germ-devouring white blood cells called leukocytes, of which 90 percent are macrophages. The remaining cells are lymphocytes composed of neutrophils and monocytes.[7] These cells are known to be non-specific immune defenders, which are involved in the ingestion and dissolution of pathogenic bacteria. They perform this immune defense work in conjunction with a group of serum proteins known as complement. There is evidence that colostrum milk can synthesize certain components of complement (called C3) and may also produce lysozyme and lactoferrin, an enzyme and a protein that have proven bactericidal effectiveness against various harmful bacteria.[8]

Intestinal Flora of Breast-Fed Infants

One of the major reasons for the substantially lower incidence of infant diarrhea in breast-fed babies is the quality of their intestinal flora. In contrast, infants who are reared on cows'-milk-based formulas have an intestinal flora that is predominantly bacteroides, streptococcus faecalis, and E. coli organisms.[9] The gut flora of exclusively breast-fed infants is colonized almost entirely with friendly bacteria: lactobacilli and bifido-bacteria.[10] In 1953, Gyorgy demonstrated that human milk contained a carbohydrate known as the bifidus factor, which may encourage the growth of these beneficial organisms.[11] In breast-fed infants, the production of ascetic acid and lactic acid by friendly lactobacillus bacteria lowers the ph (acid-alkaline balance) of the stool, thus providing a suitable acid environment, which prevents the growth of yeasts, shigella, and E. coli bacteria.[12] As a result, breast-fed infants are largely protected from the organisms associated with candida albicans, dysentery, infantile diarrhea, and gastroenteritis.

Protection Against Infant Diarrhea

In 1906 Newman reported that mortality from infant diarrhea in England was six times greater in infants receiving cows' milk formulas than those who were breast-fed.[13] This finding was far from an isolated report. In 1951, other studies by Robinson, involving 3,226 British children, revealed that the number of illnesses and deaths of infants was highest in bottle-fed babies.[14]

In some countries of Central America, where sanitation is poor and overall hygiene less than desired, breast milk has continued to prevent, to a great degree, intestinal infections in newborns. In the 1950s, studies in Guatemala (a culture where breast-feeding dominates) of Mayan women and their infants demonstrated that intestinal infections such as shigellosis (dysentery) were rare in breast-fed infants during the first few months of life.[15]

Anti-Infective Properties

Many substances in breast milk are responsible for its bactericidal and antiviral properties. Lysozyme, an enzyme found in tears and other secretions, is 300 times more concentrated in breast milk than in cows' milk.[16] Adinolfi demonstrated that lysozyme, in conjunction with complement and secretory IgA, was responsible for the dissolution of pathogenic E. coli.[17] Vitamin C (ascorbic acid) and hydrogen peroxide, which are also found in breast milk, are bactericidal against salmonella bacteria.[18] Lactoferrin, a protein found in breast milk, has a proven record of inhibiting the growth of staphylococcus aureus, E. coli, and candida albicans organisms.[19] Because lactoferrin is an iron-binding compound, it is thought to inhibit the growth of pathogenic organisms by seizing the iron necessary for their growth. Lactoperoxidase, an enzyme found in breast milk and saliva, in conjunction with hydrogen peroxide, is bactericidal against streptococci, E. coli, and salmonella organisms.

Protection From Viruses

The best protection a newborn infant has against viruses is acquired from its mother—largely from secretory IgA immunoglobulin in colostrum and mature breast milk. The production of this antibody begins during the second half of pregnancy and continues through birth and throughout the entire period the mother produces breast milk. The other protective factors in human breast milk that are effective against viruses are provided by unsaturated fatty acids (lipids), macromolecules, and active milk cells (macrophages and leukocytes).[20]

Breast Milk Kills Polio Virus

Some of the first studies that demonstrated the anti-viral activity of human milk and cows' milk against polio virus were performed by Albert Sabin and Harold Fieldsteel between 1949 and 1952.[21] Coincidentally, Albert Sabin achieved great fame when his "live" polio vaccine was introduced in 1961, replacing Salk's "killed" polio vaccine as the polio vaccine of choice. In one experiment, Sabin and Fieldsteel gathered seventy-one mothers from the greater Cincinnati, Ohio, area to test the ability of their breast milk to inactivate polio virus type 2 (Lansing strain) in mice. The colostrum milk that was drawn two to six days postpartum had an 84 percent success rate in neutralizing polio virus.[22] Even late breast milk that was drawn six to twelve months postpartum had a 73 percent neutralizing effect on the polio virus.[23] Interestingly, all the mothers whose milk exhibited anti-poliomyelitic activity had antibody to polio virus in their blood serum, though there was no corresponding relationship between the amounts of antibody in the breast milk and the serum. The seven mothers who had no polio antibody in their blood serum had no anti-polio activity in their milk.[24] Cows' milk and serum also exhibited anti-viral activity against polio virus. However, the mothers who possessed specific antibodies in their serum against herpes simplex virus did not have specific antibodies in their milk to herpes simplex—yet the breast milk neutralized herpes simplex virus! Moreover, the colostrum and breast milk also neutralized a great many other viruses with varying degrees of success, including: Japanese B encephalitis, St. Louis encephalitis, West Nile, dengue, yellow fever, and Western equine encephalitis, again with no corresponding evidence that antibodies to these viruses were in the blood serum of the mothers.[25]

These studies elucidate that human colostrum and mature breast milk, produced in lactating mothers two days to twelve months after delivery, have a very strong anti-viral activity against polio virus. They also demonstrate that breast milk has an anti-viral activity against many other viruses, independent of the presence of antibody to that virus in blood. The authors concluded that there are perhaps five other anti-viral factors in breast milk responsible for the strong anti-viral activity.[26]

Maximizing the Health of Infants

Breast-feeding is the single most important contribution a mother can make toward maximizing the health of her infant. The nutrients and immunoglobulins in breast milk will protect the baby from allergies, respiratory ailments, and childhood diseases better than anything else available.

There is nothing more joyful, more bonding, or more beautiful to the human eye than the love that is shared between a mother, a father, and their infant. Breast-feeding creates a shared intimacy between a mother and her infant that insures that the baby will get at least some of the nurturing it so desperately needs for its healthy emotional development. The art of breast-feeding and a shared intimacy between a mother, father, and their newborn is the best prescription I know of for giving infants protection against disease, and the best start possible for an emotionally rewarding life.

CHAPTER 16

An Open Letter to Parents

*E*ach year millions of parents bring their children to doctors' offices and public health clinics to be vaccinated. Most physicians believe they are doing the right thing by vaccinating babies. In my opinion, vaccination is a medical practice fraught with dangerous consequences and risks not worth taking. Injecting billions of dead bacteria or weakened living viruses preserved in hazardous chemicals into a healthy child is a reprehensible and unforgivable act. If vaccination were some sort of harmless medical procedure that did not inflict pain, create new disease syndromes, or injure and kill children, one might consider it. It is one of the great mysteries, then, that a medical procedure that has caused so much human suffering could have survived intact for so many years.

Because of vaccination's long-standing place in the history of medicine as a great medical discovery, it has been guarded and fiercely defended by most physicians and medical societies. Vaccination statutes in every state have given health departments the power and authority to demand that all children be vaccinated before they can legally attend school. With such a strong medical backing and legal precedent to support it, vaccination has set the stage for a solid and powerful business enterprise to emerge. Since the 1950s drug companies have made hundreds of millions of dollars profit from vaccines. Physicians have also reaped rewards from the overflow of consumers lining up at their doors for an ever-increasing number of vaccination shots and office visits—and with a guarantee of repeat business.

While the medical establishment does not deny that mishaps or deaths occasionally occur following the use of a vaccine, they regard these accidents as extremely rare events. Some physicians still view serious accidents, even deaths, that follow hours or days after vaccination as not being attributable to the vaccine. In any case, they say it is the price we have to pay for such a great medical invention, though imperfect, that has saved so many from serious disease and has been responsible for the decline and elimination of smallpox, diphtheria, and polio during the twentieth century. I have yet to hear a more fanciful lie.

No one knows the true number of adverse vaccine reactions. One thing is certain, however; only a small percentage of them (perhaps a third or less) have been reported. Until recently physicians were not pressured or required to report adverse vaccine reactions. Over the years, of course, many physicians have reported serious vaccine injuries to the Centers for Disease Control. There are well over two hundred articles in medical journals, published during the last seventy years, that document adverse reactions such as paralysis, meningitis, cerebral palsy, multiple sclerosis, brain damage, or seizures following the use of vaccines and serums. These journal articles have been authored almost entirely by and for physicians and medical research scientists. Much of what they have discovered about vaccines is buried in technical language and rarely reaches public view. While most of the articles are well done and brimming with scientific data, they are difficult to read and desperately lacking personal feeling. I cannot remember reading one medical journal author, whose research confirmed that vaccines were either associated with or direct causes of serious health conditions or deaths, who had the gumption to speak out against them.

In general, adverse vaccine reactions remain out of the public spotlight. However, this has not always been the case. During the 1950s, the Salk polio vaccine drew national attention after hundreds of children and adults got paralytic polio from the vaccine. In the 1960s an unknown amount of children suffered neurological disorders from the killed measles vaccine. The vaccine was such a failure that the medical profession banned it in 1967. In the 1970s, hundreds of people (and perhaps many more) suffered Guillain-Barré syndrome (and some deaths) following a mass inoculation with a flu vaccine. In the 1980s increasing numbers of infants and children suffered high-pitched screaming episodes, convulsive seizures, and collapse following the administration of the DPT vaccine. However, no matter what level of human catastrophe results from mass vaccination programs in our society, the event is quickly forgotten.

Vaccines are drugs that carry no guarantee of safety from their manufacturers. They have many documented adverse side effects. These adverse reactions, along with vaccine contraindications, are printed in the vaccine package inserts that come with the vaccine. Parents can find this detailed information in any copy of the *Physicians Desk Manual* or by asking their physician for the vaccine package insert. The vaccine information booklets that are currently distributed in clinics and pediatricians' offices and must be made available to parents prior to the administration of a vaccine explain the advantages and risks of vaccines. These booklets completely downplay the risks of vaccination and do not offer parents a viable alternative in its place. In my opinion, the information in the hand-outs, written at a sixth grade level, is a watered-down version of the facts and is neither comprehensive nor reliable enough for parents to make an informed decision on childhood immunization.

We have been led to believe that vaccination is necessary to protect children from certain childhood diseases. This is a fallacy. What we really need to do is trust in nature—and the inherent powers of disease protection that we were given at birth. Healthy newborns don't need vaccines. They need their mothers' breast milk to give them the tangible immunological resources to overcome the threat of infections. Unhealthy babies or babies with an already weakened immunity don't need vaccines because it is always questionable whether such infants can handle the overload vaccines place on their system. Sickly babies, especially ones who have no mothers to nurse them, need a great deal of loving touch and a rich supply of vitamins, minerals, and other nutrients to help build a new level of disease-protection in their little bodies. Disease organisms associated with colds, respiratory disorders, and diarrhea have a much tougher time gaining control in an infant whose gastrointestinal tract is lined with friendly, healthy bacteria supplied by breast milk.

We need to build immunity in our bodies in stages, much like the natural progression of life itself. Children accomplish this on a daily basis as they encounter, resist, fall prey to, and successfully overcome potentially dangerous organisms in their inner and outer environment. Therefore, the best thing we can do for the health of our children is to breast-feed them as infants, continue to give them healthy nourishing food as children, and make sure that they get a consistent supply of love and affection.

As I glanced through old medical books and saw pictures of the moribund bodies of infants, whose arms, buttocks, and legs became a spreading and sloughing mass of gangrenous tissue or whose skin became infested with large, spreading pustules, after smallpox vaccine went haywire inside their bodies and killed them, I felt a rage inside me that would not be silenced. After I spoke with parents whose once healthy infants became brain-damaged or killed after one or more DPT shots, a hurtful sadness filled my being. How many permanent injuries and deaths will it take to convince the American people that vaccines are an incredibly flawed and dangerous drug? How many precious infants and children need to be brain damaged or killed before an unenlightened medical profession has the courage and humanity to face the terrible truth it must eventually face?

I intended from the outset to examine the advantages and disadvantages of childhood vaccination. Certainly, there is more than one point of view about vaccination. After examining the subject in some detail, however, I see no advantage in immunization. What advantage is it to give an infant an artificial immunity of questionable value and duration, when our own natural immunity and nutritional resources are sufficient, and are unmatched by anything science could possibly invent? What statistical advantage do the vaccinated have over the unvaccinated when one-third to one-half of all reported inoculable childhood disease occurs in vaccinated individuals? And finally, how responsible an act is it for physicians to give infants hazardous chemical substances in the form of childhood vaccines when these substances have consistently caused paralysis, brain damage, a host of other syndromes and death, in a percentage of children, since the 1940s? Vaccines cannot be both protectors and destroyers of health.

Childhood vaccination is an issue of the utmost importance, and every parent should give it the consideration it deserves. In the past, many of us let that decision be made for us by physicians whose knowledge of the subject was somewhat deficient. The decision to vaccinate or not to vaccinate is yours—and yours alone to make. I hope these writings will help you to choose wisely and lead you to what is best for your child.

Sources of information in Table 14-1, provided by state health departments in letters to the author.

1. ARIZONA
   Lawrence Sands, D.O., Office of Infectious Disease Services, Arizona Department of Health Services, Phoenix, Arizona, July 24, 1990.
2. CALIFORNIA
   David S. Brown, Department of Health Services, Berkeley, California, September 14, 1990.
3. COLORADO
   Colorado Department of Health, Denver, Colorado, July 14, 1990.
4. FLORIDA
   Henry T. Janowski, M.P.H., Disease Control and AIDS Prevention, Department of Health and Rehabilitative Service, Tallahassee, Florida, July 27, 1990.
5. HAWAII
   Thomas W. Hicks, Hawaii Immunization Program, Department of Health, Honolulu, Hawaii, July 12, 1990.
6. ILLINOIS
   Robert H. Barger, Immunization Program, Department of Health, Springfield, Illinois, July 18, 1990.
7. INDIANA
   Morris Green, M.D., State Health Commissioner, Indiana State Board of Health, Indianapolis, Indiana, July 25, 1990.
8. IOWA
   Iowa Department of Public Health, Division of Disease Prevention, Des Moines, Iowa, July 12, 1990.
9. KENTUCKY
   Joe Bronowski, Manager, Immunization Program, Department for Health Service, Frankfort, Kentucky, August 6, 1990.
10. MARYLAND
    Ebenezer Israel, M.D., M.P.H., Epidemiology and Disease Control Program, Department of Health and Mental Hygiene, Baltimore, Maryland, July 20, 1990.
11. MASSACHUSETTS
    Paul Etkind, M.P.H., Division of Epidemiology, Department of Public Health, Center of Disease Control, Boston, Massachusetts, July 25, 1990.
12. MISSISSIPPI
    Brad Prescott, Immunization Program, Mississippi State Department of Health, Jackson, Mississippi, July 24, 1990.
13. MISSOURI
    Christine Mueller, Bureau of Immunization, Missouri Department of Health, Jefferson City, Missouri, July 12, 1990.

14. NEVADA
    Myla C. Florence, Administrator, Department of Human Resources, Health Division, Carson City, Nevada, July 13, 1990.
15. NEW HAMPSHIRE
    Kenneth Sharp, Immunization Program, Bureau of Disease Control, Public Health Services, Concord, New Hampshire, July 10, 1990.
16. NEW JERSEY
    C. Rod Armstrong, Immunization Program, Department of Health, Trenton, New Jersey, August 15, 1990.
17. NORTH DAKOTA
    Del Carvell, Immunization Program, Division of Disease Control, State Department of Health, Bismarck, North Dakota, July 10, 1990.
18. OHIO
    Thomas J. Halpin, M.D., M.P.H., Bureau of Preventive Medicine, Department of Health, Columbus, Ohio, July 17, 1990.
19. PENNSYLVANIA
    Phil Caves, Immunization Program, Department of Health, Harrisburg, Pennsylvania, July 16, 1990.
20. TENNESSEE
    Robert E. Flye, Department of Health and Environment, Nashville, Tennessee, July 25, 1990.
21. TEXAS
    Robert D. Crider, Jr., Immunization Division, Texas Department of Health, Austin, Texas, July 13, 1990.
22. UTAH
    Randy Tanner, Immunization Program, Department of Health, Division of Community Health Services, Salt Lake City, Utah, July 20, 1990.
23. VERMONT
    Cara M. Bryce, Immunization Technician, Department of Health, Burlington, Vermont, July 12, 1990.
24. VIRGINIA
    James B. Farrell, Bureau of Immunization, Department of Health, Richmond, Virginia, July 11, 1990.
25. WASHINGTON
    Barbara J. Baker, Office of Immunization and TB Services, Department of Health, Olympia, Washington, July 16, 1990.

Chapter 2
The Power of Human Immunity

1. *The New Encyclopaedia Brittanica*, 15th ed., s.v. "infectious diseases."
2. Ibid.
3. Ibid.
4. Ibid.
5. Ibid.
6. Ibid.
7. Mark Bricklin, *The Practical Encyclopedia of Natural Healing* (Emmaus, Pennsylvania: Rodale Press, 1983), p. 361.
8. Ivan Roitt, *Essential Immunology*, 2nd ed. (Oxford: Blackwell Scientific Publications, 1971), p. 159.
9. Bricklin, p. 361.
10. *The New Encyclopaedia Brittanica*, s.v. "infectious diseases."
11. *The New Encyclopaedia Brittanica*, s.v. "disease."
12. *The New Encyclopaedia Brittanica*, s.v. "immunity."
13. *The New Encyclopaedia Brittanica*, s.v. "infectious diseases."
14. Bricklin, p. 365.
15. *The New Encyclopaedia Brittanica*, s.v. "infectious diseases."
16. *The New American Pocket Medical Dictionary*, 13th ed., s.v. "candida."
17. "Superficial Fungal Infections," in *The Merck Manual*, 15th ed., (Rahway: Merck Sharp and Dohme Research Laboratories, 1987), p. 2270.
18. Bricklin, p. 365.
19. B.M. Greenwood, "The Host's Response to Infection," in *Oxford Textbook of Medicine*, 2nd. ed., vol. 1 (New York: Oxford University Press, 1987), sec. 5.3.
20. *Butterworths Medical Dictionary*, 2nd. ed., s.v. "antibodies."
21. Greenwood, sec. 5.3.
22. Jan Klein, *Immunology: The Science of Self-Non Self Discrimination* (New York: John Wiley and Sons, 1982), p. 516.
23. David Kingsley, *Student Microbiology Workbook* (Batavia: Genesee College Press, 1979), p. 269.
24. Roitt, p. 160-61.
25. Ibid.
26. Bricklin, p. 368.
27. Kingsley, pp. 262, 287.
28. *The New Encyclopaedia*, s.v. "immunity."
29. Ibid.
30. Ibid.
31. Roitt, p. 116.
32. Bricklin, p. 366.

33. Kingsley, p. 274.
34. Ibid., p. 275.
35. Lawrence Badgley, *Healing AIDS Naturally* (San Bruno: Human Energy Press, 1987), p. 13.
36. Ibid.
37. *The New Encyclopaedia*, s.v. "immunity."
38. Kingsley, p. 289.
39. Ibid., p. 290.
40. Ibid.
41. Badgley, p. 17.
42. Ibid., p. 18.
43. Roitt, p. 1.

Chapter 3
Immunization Versus Natural Immunity

1. Cited in Richard Moskowitz, "The Case Against Immunizations," *Journal of the American Institute of Homeopathy* 76 (1983): 14.
2. Ibid.
3. Ibid.
4. Ibid.
5. Ibid., pp. 14-15.
6. Ibid.
7. Robert Weibel et al., "Persistence of Antibody in Human Subjects for 7 to 10 Years Following Administration of Combined Live Attenuated Measles, Mumps, and Rubella Virus Vaccines," Proceedings of the Society of Experimental Biology and Medicine 165 (1980): 260-63.
8. Tracy Gustafson et al., "Measles Outbreak in a Fully Immunized Secondary-School Population," *New England Journal of Medicine* 316, no. 13 (1987): 771.
9. B.M. Greenwood, "The Host's Response to Infection," in *Oxford Textbook of Medicine*, 2nd ed., vol. 1 (New York: Oxford University Press, 1987), sec. 5.3.
10. Cited in Harold Buttram and John Chriss Hoffman, *Vaccinations and Immune Malfunction* (Quakertown: The Randolph Society, 1985), p. 22.
11. Buttram and Hoffman, p. 22.
12. Ibid.
13. Recommendations of the Immunization Practices Advisory Committee (ACIP). *MMWR* 1991; 40 (No.RR-12):56.
14. F.M. Burnett, *The Integrity of the Body* (Cambridge: Harvard University Press, 1962), p. 173.
15. Julian Davies and Barbara Shaffer Littlewood, *Elementary Biochemistry: An Introduction to the Chemistry of Living Cells* (Englewood Cliffs: Prentice-Hall, 1979), p. 288.

16. Ibid.
17. Ibid., p. 293.
18. Ibid.
19. Ibid.
20. Ibid., p. 294.
21. Jan Klein, *Immunology: The Science of Self-Non Self Discrimination* (New York: John Wiley and Sons, 1982), p. 600.
22. Cited in Moskowitz, p. 16.
23. Ibid.
24. Moskowitz, p. 16.

Chapter 4
The Making of a Vaccine

1. A.J. Beale, "Vaccines and Antiviral Drugs" in *Topley and Wilson's Principles of Bacteriology, Virology and Immunity*, 7th ed., vol. 4 (Baltimore: Williams and Wilkins, 1984), p. 149.
2. V.A. Jegede et al., "Vaccine Technology," in *Encyclopedia of Chemical Technology*, 3rd. ed., (New York: John Wiley and Sons, 1983), p. 629.
3. Ibid., pp. 628-29.
4. Jegede et al., p. 630.
5. Ibid.
6. *The New Encyclopaedia Brittanica*, 15th ed., s.v. "industries, chemical process."
7. Sir Graham Wilson, *The Hazards of Immunization* (London: The Athlone Press, 1967), p. 19.
8. Jegede et al., p. 630.
9. *The New Encyclopaedia Brittanica*, s.v. "industries, chemical process."
10. Jegede et al., p. 630.
11. Ibid., p. 631.
12. Ibid.
13. Ibid.
14. Harris Coulter and Barbara Loe Fisher, *DPT: A Shot in the Dark* (New York: Harcourt Brace Jovanovich, 1985), p. 28.
15. 21 C.F.R. sec. 600.4 (1990).
16. Ibid.
17. Ibid.
18. Ibid.
19. 21 C.F.R. sec. 600.5 (1990).
20. Ibid.
21. Coulter and Fisher, p. 28.

Chapter 5
Vaccination and Animal Experimentation

1. Ed Harlow and David Lane, *Antibodies: A Laboratory Manual* (Cold Spring Harbor: Cold Spring Harbor Laboratories, 1988), p. 93.

2. Harold Johnson and Charles Leach, "Studies On The Single Injection Method Of Canine Rabies Vaccination," *American Journal of Public Health* 32 (1942): 176-177.

3. Coenraad Henricksen, *Laboratory Animals in Vaccine Production and Control* (Norwell, Massachusetts: Kluwer Academic Publishers, 1988), pp. 37-41.

4. Ibid.

5. Peter Singer, *Animal Liberation* (New York: New York Review of Books, 1975), p. 48.

6. Ibid.

7. Ibid., p. 49.

8. Ibid.

9. Singer, p. 28.

10. Ibid., p. 29.

11. Ibid.

12. Richard Egdahl, "Chronic Uncontrolled Cross-Circulation in Unanesthetized Dogs," *Science* 122 (1955): 245-46.

13. J.S. Younger, Elsie Ward, and Jonas Salk, "Studies on Poliomyelitis Viruses in Cultures of Monkey Testicular Tissue," *American Journal of Hygiene* 55 (1952): 292.

14. Ibid.

15. Ibid.

16. Ibid., p. 292-93.

17. Ibid.

18. Ibid., p. 294.

19. Ibid.

20. Cited in Younger, Ward, and Salk, p. 291.

21. Younger, Ward, and Salk, p. 294.

22. A.J. Beale, "Vaccines and Antiviral Drugs," in *Topley and Wilson's Principles of Bacteriology, Virology and Immunity*, 7th ed., vol. 4 (Baltimore: Williams and Wilkins, 1984), p. 151.

23. Sir Graham Wilson, *The Hazards of Immunization* (London: The Athlone Press, 1967), p. 56.

24. Ibid.

25. Ibid., p. 57.

26. Beale, p. 151.

27. Wilson, p. 55.

28. Beale, p. 151.

29. Ibid., p. 153.
30. Ibid., p. 151.
31. Wilson, p. 139.
32. Ibid., p. 140.
33. Ibid., pp. 139-40.
34. Ibid., p. 141.
35. Ferdinand Kojis, "Serum Sickness and Anaphylaxis," *American Journal of Diseases of Children* 64 (1942): 93, 213.
36. *The Vaccination Inquirer*, vol. 94, no. 909, cited in Elben, *Vaccination Condemned* (Los Angeles: Better Life Research, 1981), p. 286-87.
37. "What is Pure Lymph?," *Westminster Review* 165, no. 3 (1906): 311.
38. Francis Martin, *"The Propagation, Preservation, and Use of Vaccine Virus"* (New York: The Publishers' Printing Company, 1896), pp. 6-9.

Chapter 6
Witch's Brew: Toxic Chemicals in Vaccines

1. H.M. Powell and W.A. Jamieson, "Merthiolate as a Germicide," *American Journal of Hygiene* 13 (1931): 296.
2. Ibid., p. 299.
3. Ibid.
4. Ibid.
5. Ibid., p. 304.
6. Ibid.
7. Ibid., p. 305.
8. Ibid., p. 307.
9. Ibid., p. 306.
10. Ibid., p. 309.
11. Harry Morton, Leon North, and Frank Engley, "The Bacteriostatic and Bactericidal Actions of Some Mercurial Compounds on Hemolytic Streptococci," *Journal of the American Medical Association* 136, no. 1 (1948): 40.
12. Ibid.
13. Ibid.
14. Philip Price, "The Meaning of Bacteriostasis, Bactericidal Effect, and Rate of Disinfection," *Annals of the New York Academy of Sciences* 53 (1950): 78-79.
15. Ibid.
16. Edwin Davisson et al., "The Preservation of Poliomyelitis Vaccine with Stabilized Merthiolate," *Journal of Laboratory and Clinical Medicine* 47 (1956): 15.
17. Ibid.
18. Ibid., p. 14.

19. Ibid., p. 18.

20. Henry Welch and Albert Hunter, "Method for Determining the Effect of Chemical Antisepsis on Phagocytosis," *American Journal of Public Health* 30 (1940): 129.

21. Ibid., p. 130.

22. Ibid., p. 132.

23. Ibid., p. 135.

24. Ibid.

25. Ibid., p. 136.

26. Ibid.

27. Cited in Morton, North, and Engley, p. 41.

28. Ibid.

29. Ibid.

30. Robert Waller, "The Action of Sodium Ethylmercurithiosalicylate on Human Anti-Rh Serums," *American Journal of Clinical Pathology* 8 (1944): 116-17.

31. Morton, North, and Engley, p. 41.

32. M.R. Haeney et al., "Long-Term Parenteral Exposure to Mercury in Patients with Hypogammaglobulinaemia," *British Medical Journal* 2 (1979): 12.

33. Cited in Haeney et al., p. 14.

34. David Matheson, Thomas Clarkson, and Erwin Gelfand, "Mercury Toxicity (Acrodynia) Induced by Long-Term Injection of Gammaglobulin," *Journal of Pediatrics* 97, no. 1 (1980): 153.

35. Cited in Morton, North, and Engley, p. 41.

36. *Casarett and Doull's Toxicology, The Basic Science of Poisons*, 3rd. ed. Curtis Klaassen, Mary Amdur, John Doull eds., (New York: MacMillan Publishing Company, 1986), pp. 422-23.

37. Ibid.

38. Ibid.

39. Michael Wills and John Savory, "Aluminum Poisoning: Dialysis Encephalopathy, Osteomalacia, and Anaemia," *Lancet* (July 2, 1983): 29.

40. Cited in Wills and Savory, p. 30.

41. Ibid.

42. Ibid.

43. Ibid.

44. Ibid.

45. Harris Coulter and Barbara Loe Fisher, *DPT: A Shot in the Dark* (New York: Harcourt Brace Jovanovich, 1985) p. 25.

46. Jan Klein, *Immunology: The Science of Self-Non Self Discrimination* (New York: John Wiley and Sons, 1982), p. 361.

47. Ibid., p. 362.

48. Ibid., p. 361.

49. O. Kohashi et al., "Effect of Oil Composition on Both Adjuvant-Induced Arthritis and Delayed Hypersensitivity Derivatives and Peptidoglycans in Various Rat Strains," *Infection and Immunity* 17, no. 2 (1977): 244.

50. W. Henle and G. Henle, "Effect of Adjuvants on Vaccination of Human Beings Against Influenza," *Proceedings of the Society for Experimental Biology and Medicine* 59 (1945): 181.

51. Carl Pearson, "Development of Arthritis Periarthritis and Periostitis In Rats Given Adjuvants," *Proceedings of the Society for Experimental Biology and Medicine* 91 (1956): 95-101.

52. B. Waksman, C.M. Pearson, and J.T. Sharp, "Studies of Arthritis and Other Lesions Induced in Rats by Injection of Mycobacterial Adjuvant," *Journal of Immunology* 85 (1960): 416.

53. J.A. Bell et al., "Epidemiologic Studies on Influenza in Familial And General Population Groups, 1951-1956. IV. Vaccine Reactions," *American Journal of Hygiene* 73 (1961): 155.

54. Ibid.

55. *The New American Pocket Medical Dictionary*, 13th ed., s.v. "granuloma."

56. Bell et al., p. 155.

57. Ibid., p. 157.

58. Ibid., p. 168.

59. Ibid., p. 161.

60. Ibid., p. 160.

61. Cited in Robert Mendelsohn, *The Risks of Immunization and How To Avoid Them* (Evanston: The People's Doctor, Inc., 1988), p. 8.

62. E. Harlow and D. Lane, *Antibodies: A Laboratory Manual* (Cold Spring Harbor: Cold Spring Harbor Laboratory, 1988), p. 99.

63. Robert Gosselin, Roger Smith, and Harold Hodge, *Clinical Toxicology of Commercial Products*, 5th ed., (Baltimore: Williams and Wilkins, 1984), sec. III-196.

64. Marshall Sittig, *Handbook of Toxic and Hazardous Chemicals and Carcinogens*, 2nd ed., (Park Ridge, New Jersey: Noyes Publications, 1985), p. 462.

65. Harris and Fisher, p. 23.

66. Gosselin, Smith, and Hodge, sec. III-197.

67. Ibid.

68. Ibid.

69. Ibid., sec. III-196.

70. Ibid.

71. Sittig, p. 462.

72. Gosselin, Smith, and Hodge, sec. III-197.

73. Ibid.

74. Klaassen, Amdur, and Doull, eds., p. 819.

75. M.V. Veldee, "Regarding Salk Vaccine," *New England Journal of Medicine* 252, no. 11 (1955): 483.
76. Ibid.
77. Sir Graham Wilson, *The Hazards of Immunization* (London: The Athlone Press, 1967), p. 46.
78. Ibid.
79. Ibid.
80. Neal Nathanson and Alexander Langmuir, "The Cutter Incident. Poliomyelitis Following Formaldehyde-Inactivated Poliovirus Vaccination in the United States during the Spring of 1955, " *American Journal of Hygiene* 78 (1963): 39.
81. Ibid.
82. Wilson, p. 47.
83. Marcus Mason, C.C. Cate, and John Baker, "Toxicology and Carcinogenesis of Various Chemicals Used in The Preparation of Vaccines," *Clinical Toxicology* 4 (1971): 185.
84. Ibid., p. 194.
85. Ibid.
86. Ibid., p. 203.
87. Ibid., p. 200.
88. Ibid., p. 197.
89. Ibid., p. 201.

Chapter 7
The Provocation Effect of Vaccines and Other Drugs

1. J. Trueta and R. Hodes, "Provoking And Localizing Factors In Poliomyelitis," *Lancet* 1 (1954): 998-99.
2. Ibid.
3. Ibid.
4. Ibid.
5. Ibid., p. 1000.
6. Ibid.
7. Cited in Sir Graham Wilson, *The Hazards of Immunization* (London: The Athlone Press, 1967), p. 277.
8. Wilson, p. 272.
9. Cited in Wilson, p. 272.
10. Wilson, p. 273.
11. Ibid., p. 274.
12. Russel Schaedler and René Dubos, "Effects of Cellular Constituents Of Mycobacteria on The Resistance of Mice to Heterologous Infections," *Journal of Experimental Medicine* 106 (1957): 726.

13. Wilson, p. 277.

14. Ibid., p. 279.

15. Ralph Scobey, "The Poison Cause of Poliomyelitis and Obstructions to Its Investigation," *Archives of Pediatrics* 69 (1952): 172-73.

Chapter 8
The Decline of Childhood Diseases Before Vaccination

1. Louis Dublin and Alfred Lotka, *Twenty-Five Years of Health Progress* (New York: Metropolitan Life Insurance Company, 1937), p. 48.

2. Ibid., p. 45.

3. Louis Dublin, *Health Progress 1936-1945* (New York: Metropolitan Life Insurance Company, 1948), p. 12.

4. Dublin and Lotka, p. 63.

5. Ibid., p. 65.

6. Ibid.

7. Ibid.

8. George Bigelow, *Report of the Committee on Communicable Disease Control* (New York: The Century Company, 1931), p. 145.

9. Ibid., p. 144.

10. Dublin and Lotka, p. 67.

11. Ibid., p. 70.

12. Dublin, p. 18.

13. Dublin and Lotka, p. 75.

14. Ibid.

15. Ibid., p. 76.

16. Harris Coulter and Barbara Loe Fisher, *DPT: A Shot in the Dark* (New York: Harcourt Brace Jovanovich, 1985), p. 19.

17. Ibid.

18. Ibid.

19. Dublin and Lotka, p. 56.

20. Ibid., p. 58.

21. Ibid., p. 59.

22. Ibid., p. 60.

23. Ibid., p. 58.

24. Ibid.

25. *The New Encyclopaedia Brittanica*, 15th ed., s.v. "infectious disease."

26. Sir Graham Wilson, *The Hazards of Immunization* (London: The Athlone Press, 1967), p. 21-22.

27. Ibid., p. 38.

Chapter 9
Whooping Cough In Vaccinated and Unvaccinated Children

1. Edgar Sydenstricker and Ralph Wheeler, "Whooping Cough in Surveyed Communities," *American Journal of Public Health* 26 (1936): 576-77.
2. Ibid.
3. Ibid.
4. *Mortality Statistics* (Washington, D.C.: United States Department of Commerce, Bureau of Census, 1933), p. 6.
5. George Bigelow, *Report of the Committee on Communicable Disease Control* (New York: The Century Company, 1931), p. 211.
6. Ibid., p. 24.
7. Ibid., p. 211.
8. James Doull, Gerald Shibley, and Joseph McClelland, "Active Immunization Against Whooping Cough," *American Journal of Public Health* 26 (1936): 1100-01.
9. Ibid.
10. Ibid., p. 1105.
11. James Perkins et al., "Field Study of the Prophylactic Value of Pertussis Vaccine," *American Journal of Public Health* 32 (1942): 63.
12. Ibid., p. 69.
13. Ibid.
14. Ibid., p. 70.
15. A.M. McFarlan, E. Topley, and M. Fisher, "Trial Of Whooping Cough Vaccine in City and Residential Nursery Groups," *British Medical Journal* (August 18, 1945): 207-208.
16. Gordon Stewart, "Vaccination Against Whooping-Cough, Efficacy Versus Risks," *Lancet* (January 29, 1977): 234.
17. Ibid., p. 235.
18. Ibid., p. 235.
19. Ibid.
20. Ibid., p. 236.
21. Paul Fine and Jacqueline Clarkson, "The Recurrence Of Whooping Cough: Possible Implications for Assessment of Vaccine Efficacy," *Lancet* (March 20, 1982): 668.
22. Ibid.
23. Stephen Palmer, "Vaccine Efficacy and Control Measures in Pertussis," *Archives of Disease in Childhood* 66 (1991): 854.
24. Fine and Clarkson, p. 667.
25. Ibid.
26. Ibid., p. 666.
27. John Taranger, "Mild Clinical Course of Pertussis in Swedish Infants of Today," *Lancet* (June 12, 1982): 1360.

28. Ibid.
29. Harris Coulter and Barbara Loe Fisher, *DPT: A Shot in the Dark* (New York: Harcourt Brace Jovanovich, 1985), p. 172.
30. Taranger, p. 1360.
31. Coulter and Fisher, p. 163.
32. Vincent Fulginiti, "Controversies in Current Immunization Policy and Practices: One Physician's Viewpoint," *Current Problems in Pediatrics* 6 (1976): 8.
33. Ibid.

Chapter 10
The Adverse Reactions To Vaccines

1. Tracy Gustafson et al., "Measles Outbreak in a Fully Immunized Secondary-School Population," *New England Journal of Medicine* 316 (1987): 771.
2. Alexander Langmuir and Neal Nathanson, "The Cutter Incident. Poliomyelitis Following Formaldehyde-Inactivated Poliovirus Vaccination in the United States during the Spring of 1955," *American Journal of Hygiene* 78 (1963): 25, 39.
3. Harris Coulter and Barbara Loe Fisher, *DPT: A Shot in the Dark* (New York: Harcourt Brace Jovanovich, 1985), p. 53.
4. Ibid.
5. Ibid., pp. 58-59.
6. Ibid., p. 63.
7. *Pertussis and Pertussis Vaccine: Information for Parents* (Dissatisfied Parents Together, 128 Branch Road, Vienna, Virginia, 1985), p. 11.
8. Harris and Coulter, p. 69.
9. Ibid.
10. Ibid., p. 71.
11. Ibid., p. 72.
12. Ibid.
13. Ibid.
14. Ibid., p. 74.
15. Ibid., p. 75.
16. Ibid., p. 76.
17. Ibid., p. 75.
18. Ibid., p. 76.
19. Ibid.
20. Ibid., p. 245.
21. Ibid., pp. 243-45.
22. Alan Hinman and Jeffrey Koplan, "Pertussis and Pertussis Vaccine: Reanalysis of Benefits, Risks and Costs," *Journal of the American Medical Association* 251, no. 23 (1984): 3109-13.

23. Cited in Sir Graham Wilson, *The Hazards of Immunization* (London: The Athlone Press, 1967), p. 63.

24. Ibid., pp. 21-23.

25. George Wilson and Samuel Hadden, "Neuritis and Multiple Neuritis Following Serum Therapy," *Journal of the American Medical Association* 98, no. 2 (1932): 123.

26. Forrest Young, "Peripheral Nerve Paralysis Following the Use of Various Serums," *Journal of the American Medical Association* 98 (1932): 1139.

27. Thorvald Madsden, "Vaccination Against Whooping Cough," *Journal of the American Medical Association* 101 (1933): 187.

28. Ferdinand Kojis, "Serum Sickness and Anaphylaxis," *American Journal of Diseases of Children* 64 (1942): 129.

29. W. Sako et al., "Early Immunization Against Pertussis with Alum-Precipitated Vaccine," *Journal of the American Medical Association* 127 (1945): 379.

30. Richard Capps, Victor Sborov, and Charles Scheiffley, "A Syringe-Transmitted Epidemic of Infectious Hepatitis," *Journal of the American Medical Association* 136, no. 12 (1948): 819.

31. J. Werne and I. Garrow, "Fatal Anaphylactic Shock Occurrence in Identical Twins Following Second Injection of Diphtheria Toxoid and Pertussis Antigen," *Journal of the American Medical Association* 131, no. 9 (1946): 730-35.

32. Randolph Byers and Frederic Moll, "Encephalopathies Following Prophylactic Pertussis Vaccine," *Pediatrics* 1, no. 4 (1948): 440-41.

33. Wilson, p. 38.

34. J. Globus and J. Kohn, "Encephalopathy Following Pertussis Vaccine Prophylaxis," *Journal of the American Medical Association* 141, no. 8 (1949): 507-09.

35. J. Toomey, "Reactions To Pertussis Vaccine," *Journal of the American Medical Association* 139, no. 7 (1949): 448-50.

36. S.R. Halpern and D. Halpern, "Reactions from DPT Immunization and its Relationship to Allergic Children," *Journal of Pediatrics* 47 (1955): 60-67.

37. D. Geffen, J.H. Patterson and S.M. Tracy, "Poliomyelitis Following Inoculation. A Survey of 29 Children," *Lancet* (June 27, 1953): 1269-72.

38. H.J. Miller and J.B. Stanton, "Neurologic Sequelae of Prophylactic Inoculation," *Quarterly Journal of Medicine* 89 (1954):1-27.

39. Ibid.

40. Ibid.

41. C.N. Christensen, "More Risky to Give Or Not to Give," *American Journal of Diseases of Children* 105 (1963): 417.

42. M. Kulenkampff, M. Schwartzman, and J. Wilson, "Neurological Complications of Pertussis Inoculation," *Archives of Disease in Childhood* 49 (1974): 46-49.

43. Gordon Stewart, "Vaccination Against Whooping-Cough, Efficacy Versus Risks," *Lancet* (January 29, 1977): 236.

44. A.H. Griffith, "Reactions After Pertussis Vaccine: A Manufacturer's Experiences and Difficulties Since 1964," *British Medical Journal* 1 (April 1, 1978): 809-15.

45. J. Jacob and F. Manning, "Increased Intracranial Pressure After Diphtheria, Tetanus and Pertussis Immunization," *American Journal of Diseases of Children* 133 (1979): 217-18.

46. Gordon Stewart, "Toxicity of Pertussis Vaccine: Frequency and Probability of Reactions," *Journal of Epidemiology and Community Health* 33, no. 2 (1979): 150-156.

47. W.C. Torch, "Diphtheria-Pertussis-Tetanus (DPT) Immunization: A Potential Cause of Sudden Infant Death Syndrome (SIDS)," *Neurology* 32, no. 4 (1982): Part 2.

48. Pearay Ogra and Kenneth Herd, "Arthritis Associated with Induced Rubella Infection," *Journal of Immunology* 107 (1971): 810-13.

49. Henry Miller, Wojciench Cendrowski, and Kurt Schapira, "Multiple Sclerosis and Vaccination," *British Medical Journal* 2 (1967): 210-13.

50. G.M. Findlay and F.O. MacCallum, "Hepatitis and Jaundice Associated with Immunizing Against Certain Virus Diseases," Proceedings of the Royal Society of Medicine 31 (1938): 799.

51. "Jaundice Following Yellow Fever Vaccination," (Editorial) *Journal of the American Medical Association* 119 (1942): 1110.

52. Philip Landrigan and John Witte, "Neurologic Disorders Following Live Measles-Virus Vaccination," *Journal of the American Medical Association* 223, no. 13 (1973): 1459-62.

53. P. Beeson, G. Chesney, and A.M. MacFarlan, "Hepatitis Following Injection Of Mumps Convalescent Plasma, " Lancet (June 24, 1944): 814-16.

54. "Meningitis Risk Seen from Use of Vaccine," St. Paul Pioneer Press Dispatch, April 21, 1987, p. 1A.

55. A.B. Hill and J. Knowelden, "Inoculation and Poliomyelitis. A Statistical Investigation in England and Wales in 1949," *British Medical Journal* (July 1, 1950): 1.

56. Morris Greenburg et al., "The Relation Between Recent Injection and Paralytic Poliomyelitis in Children," *American Journal of Public Health* 42 (1952): 142.

57. Report of the Medical Research Council Committee on Inoculation Procedures and Neurological Lesions. "Poliomyelitis and Prophylactic Inoculation Against Diphtheria, Whooping-Cough, and Smallpox," Lancet (December 15, 1956): 1223-1231.

58. Sir Graham Wilson, *The Hazards of Immunization* (London: The Athlone Press, 1967), pp. 160-64.

59. F. Markum et al., "Discussion on Immunization of Man Against Measles," *American Journal of Diseases of Children* 103 (1962): 390-93.

60. Ian Mair and Haus Elverland, "Sudden Deafness and Vaccination," *Journal of Laryngology and Otology*," 91 (1977): 323-29.

61. NVIC News, vol. 1, no. 3 (National Vaccine Information Center, 128 Branch Road, Vienna, Virginia, 1991), p. 3.

62. Ibid.

63. Ibid.

64. Ibid., p. 5.

65. Vaccine Injury Compensation Program, *Weekly Status Report, February 18, 1992* (Rockville, Maryland: Department of Health and Human Services, Public Health Service, Bureau of Health Professions, Health Resources and Services Administration).

Chapter 11
Measles in the 1980s

1. Measles—United States, 1990. *Morbidity and Mortality Weekly Report (MMWR)* 1991;40(2):369.

2. Measles. *MMWR* 1990;39(41):726.

3. Measles. *MMWR* 1990;39(21):362.

4. "Childhood Infections" in *The Merck Manual*, 15th ed., Robert Berkow and Andrew Fletcher, eds., (Rahway: Merck Sharp and Dohme Research Laboratories, 1987), p. 2022.

5. A.B. Block et al., "Health Impact of Measles Vaccination in the United States," *Pediatrics* 76, no.4 (1985): 525.

6. S.R. Preblud and S.L. Katz, "Measles Vaccine," in *Vaccines*, Stanley Plotkin and Edward Mortimer, eds., (Philadelphia: W.B. Saunders, 1988), p. 187.

7. Ibid.

8. Ibid., p. 190.

9. Measles—United States. *MMWR* 1977;26(14):109.

10. Ibid.

11. Ibid., p. 110.

12. National Center for Health Statistics. *Health, United States, 1989* (Hyattsville, Maryland: Public Health Service, 1990), p. 40.

13. *MMWR* 1991;40(22):370.

14. Ibid.

15. D.L. Eddins, "Indications Of Immunization Status," 17th Immunization Conference Proceedings, Public Health Service, May 18-19, 1982.

16. National Center for Health Statistics, p. 40.

17. *MMWR* 1990;39(21):354.

18. Tracy Gustafson et al., "Measles Outbreak in a Fully Immunized Secondary-School Population," *New England Journal of Medicine* 316, no.13 (1987): 771.

19. Ibid.

20. Ibid.

21. Ibid., p. 773.

22. Update: Measles Outbreak—Chicago 1989. *MMWR* 1990;39(19):318.

23. Measles—United States. *MMWR* 1977;26(14): 110.

24. Preblud and Katz, p. 196.

25. Ibid.

26. *MMWR* 1977;26(14):110.

27. Philip Landrigan and John Witte, "Neurologic Disorders Following Live Measles-Virus Vaccination," *Journal of the American Medical Association* 223, no. 13 (1973): 1460.

28. Cited in Preblud and Katz, p. 189.

29. Robert Berkow and Andrew Fletcher, eds., *The Merck Manual*, p. 1803.

30. Cited in Preblud and Katz, p. 197.

31. W. Orenstein et al., "Impact Of Revaccinating Children Who Received Vaccine Before 10 Months," *Pediatrics* 77 (1986): 474.

32. *MMWR* 1990;39(19):317.

33. H. Bigelow, *Report of the Committee on Communicable Disease Control, White House Conference on Child Health and Protection* (New York: The Century Company, 1931), p. 144.

34. Ibid.

35. G.E. Hardy, "The Failure of a School Immunization Campaign to Terminate an Urban Epidemic of Measles," *American Journal of Epidemiology* 91, no. 3 (1970): 286.

36. Ibid., pp. 286-88.

37. Ibid.

38. W.L. Carr, "A Report on Cases of Measles," *Archives of Pediatrics* 16 (1899): 1-15.

39. Ibid.

40. Bigelow, p. 144.

41. Ibid.

42. Hardy, p. 288-91.

43. Measles Vaccination Level Among Selected Groups of Preschool-Aged Children— United States. *MMWR* 1991;40(2):36-37.

44. Ibid., pp. 37-38.

45. Ibid., p. 38.

46. Edward Godfrey, "Measles in Institutions for Children," *Medical Hypothesis* 2, part 3 (1928): 272.

47. *MMWR* 1990;39(21):354.

48. Ibid., p. 355.

49. Ibid.

50. Robert Berkow and Andrew Fletcher, eds., *The Merck Manual*, p. 2023.

51. Vincent Fulginiti et al., "Altered Reactivity To Measles Virus," *Journal of the American Medical Association* 202, no. 12 (1967): 101-106.

52. Robert Berkow and Andrew Fletcher, eds., *The Merck Manual*, p. 2023.

53. Fulginiti et al., p. 106.
54. Ibid.
55. Landrigan and Witte, p. 1459.
56. Ibid., p. 1460.
57. Ibid., p. 1461.
58. Tove Ronne, "Measles Virus Infection Without Rash in Childhood Is Related to Disease in Adult Life," *Lancet* (January 5, 1985): 2-3.
59. Ibid.
60. Cited in Ronne, p. 3.
61. Ibid., pp. 2-3.
62. Ibid.
63. Ibid.
64. Ibid., p. 3.
65. *MMWR* 1990;39(41):727-28.
66. Ibid.
67. Ibid.
68. Ibid.
69. Ibid.
70. H.F. Hull et al., "Risk Factors for Measles Vaccine Failure Among Immunized Students," *Pediatrics* 76 (1985): 518-23.
71. Gustafson et al., p. 773.
72. CDC, unpublished data. *MMWR* 1990;39(19):326.
73. Vincent Fulginiti and Ray Helfer, "Atypical Measles In Adolescent Siblings 16 Years After Killed Measles Virus Vaccine," *Journal of the American Medical Association* 244, no. 8 (1980): 804.
74. Ibid.
75. Ibid., p. 805.
76. Cited in R. Moskowitz, "Immunization: The Other Side," in *Vaccinations: A Selection Of Articles, Letters and Resources 1979-1989* (Santa Fe: Mothering Magazine, 1989), p. 36.
77. Stephen Preblud and Walter Orenstein, "Chickenpox" in *Maxy-Rosenau Public Health and Preventative Medicine*, 12th ed., (Norwalk: Appelton-Century-Crofts, 1986), p. 172.
78. Ibid.
79. Ibid.
80. Ibid.
81. Ibid., p. 171.
82. Ibid., p. 172.

Chapter 12
The Myth of Vaccine Immunity

1. Leon Chaitow, *Vaccination and Immunization: Dangers, Delusions and Alternatives* (Saffron, England: C.F. Daniel Company, Ltd., 1987), pp. 41-43.

2. Percival Hartley et al., "A Study of Diphtheria in Two Areas of Great Britain," Special Report Series no. 272 (London: His Majesty's Stationery Office, 1950), pp. 65, 99-107.

3. Vincent Fulginiti, "Controversies In Current Immunization Policy and Practices: One Physicians Viewpoint," *Current Problems in Pediatrics* 6, no. 6 (1976): 14.

4. Ibid., p. 15.

5. Ibid., p. 16.

6. Ibid.

Chapter 13
Vaccination and the Law

1. Mass. Gen. L. ch. 21, sec. 42-43 (1835).

2. Mass. Gen. L. ch. 414, sec. 1-2-3 (1855).

3. *Jacobson v. Massachusetts*, 197 U. S. 11,14 (1905).

4. Id.

5. In *Jacobson v. Massachusetts* (1905) the Supreme Court examined the viability of smallpox vaccination (as a side issue) by comparing smallpox deaths in vaccinated and unvaccinated people. (See footnotes, *Jacobson v. Massachusetts*, 197 U.S. 11 at 32-34). One set of figures used in *Jacobson* and cited from *Johnson's Universal Cyclopaedia* (1897), reveal a large discrepancy between deaths in the unvaccinated (46.3%) versus those deaths in people vaccinated for smallpox (1.7%). By contrast, the noted medical historian Jurin tabulated the death-rate for smallpox to be 18.8% for the entire 18th century, or the one-hundred year period before vaccination commenced (*Encyclopaedia Brittanica*, 9th ed., "vaccination"). Likewise, during the 19th century, the death-rate from smallpox in British and American hospitals from 1870 to 1885 among the vaccinated and unvaccinated combined was 18.5% (Op. cit., p. 29). This fact (as well as many others) casts doubt upon the figures used as supplementary material in *Jacobson* and begs for the entire subject to be reconsidered. For an unbiased analysis of smallpox vaccination statistics, read the article on "vaccination" in the 9th edition of the *Encyclopaedia Brittanica* (1885).

6. *Encyclopedia Brittanica*, 9th ed., s.v. "vaccination."

7. W. Young and G. Wilkinsen, *Vaccination Tracts: Facts and Figures* (Providence: Snow and Farnum, 1892), p. 5.

8. G.F. Kolb, Royal Statistical Commission of Bavaria (in a letter to William Tebb, 22nd January, 1882) in William White, *The Story of A Great Delusion* (London: E.W. Allen, 1885), p. 596.

9. White, p. 492.
10. Tom Finn, *Dangers of Compulsory Immunization: How to Avoid Them Legally* (New Port Richey, Florida: Family Fitness Press, 1983), p. 6.
11. *Jacobson v. Massachusetts*, 197 U. S. at 13.
12. *Commonwealth v. Jacobson*, 183 Mass. 242, 246 (1904).
13. U.S. Constitution art. 14, sec. 1.
14. *Jacobson v. Massachusetts*, 197 U. S. at 17.
15. Id.
16. Id.
17. Id. at 29.
18. Id. at 34-35.
19. Id. at 39.
20. Id.
21. Finn, p. 6.
22. Cited in Finn, p. 6.

Chapter 14
How To Legally Avoid Immunization

1. J. Hale, et al., *State Immunization Requirements for School Children* (Atlanta: Centers for Disease Control, Center for Prevention Services, Immunization Division, 1981).
2. Tom Finn, *Dangers of Compulsory Immunizations: How To Avoid Them Legally* (New Port Richey, Florida: Family Fitness Press, 1983), p. 31.
3. *Parents Guide to Childhood Immunization* (Atlanta: Public Health Service, Centers for Disease Control, rev. 1988), p. 6; Recommendations of the Immunization Practices Advisory Committee (ACIP). *MMWR* 1992; 41(No.RR-1) :8-9; *Immunization of Adults: A Call to Action* (Atlanta: Public Health Service, Centers for Disease Control, rev. 1991), p. 7; Meruvax II and M-M-R II, Manufacturer's Packet Insert (West Point, Pennsylvania: Merck Sharp and Dohme, October 1986); General Recommendations on Immunization. *MMWR* 1983; 32 (No. 1); Polio Virus Vaccine Live Oral Trivalent Orimune, Sabin Strains 1, 2, and 3. Manufacturer's Packet Insert (Pearl River, New York: Lederle Laboratories, August 1986).
4. *Parents Guide to Childhood Immunization*, p. 6.
5. Table 14-1.
6. Harris Coulter and Barbara Loe Fisher, *DPT: A Shot in the Dark* (New York: Harcourt Brace Jovanovich, 1985), p. 373.
7. Ibid.
8. Ibid.
9. Mass. Gen. Laws Ann. ch. 76, sec. 15 (1983) amended by 1967 Mass. Acts c. 590, sec. 15.
10. Id.

11. *Dalli v. Board of Education*, 267 N.E.2nd 219, 358 Mass. 753,754 (1971).
12. Id. at 755.
13. Id.
14. Id. at 759.
15. Id.
16. Mass. Gen. Laws. Ann. ch. 76, sec. 15 (1983) amended by 1971 Mass. Acts. ch. 285.
17. *Dalli v. Board of Education*, 267 N.E.2nd at 758.
18. N.Y. Pub. Health Law sec. 2164(9) (McKinney 1985).
19. *Sherr v. Northport-East Northport U. Free School District*, 672 F Supp. 81 (E.D.N.Y. 1987).
20. Id. at 96.
21. Id. at 95.
22. Id.
23. Id. at 97.
24. Id.
25. Id.
26. Id. at 99. For New York's current vaccination statutes see N.Y. Pub. Health Law sec. 2164 (McKinney Supp. 1992).
27. *Mason v. General Brown Central School District*, 851 F. 2nd 47 (2nd Cir. 1988).
28. Id. at 50.
29. Ark. Code. Ann. sec. 6-18-702 (Michie 1987).
30. Colo. Rev. Stat. sec. 25-4-903 (1982).
31. Fla. Stat. Ann. sec. 232.032 (West 1989).
32. Ind. Code Ann. sec. 20-8. 1-7-2 (West 1984).
33. Mass. Ann. Laws ch. 76 sec. 15 (Law. Co-op. 1991).
34. Mich. Comp. Laws Ann. 333.9215 (West Supp. 1992).
35. N.H. Rev. Stat. Ann. sec. 141-C:20-c (1990).
36. Ohio Rev. Code Ann. sec. 3313.671 (Page 1990).
37. Tex. Educ. Code Ann. sec. 2.09 (West 1991 & Supp. 1992).
38. Wis. Stat. Ann. sec. 140.05 (West 1989 & Supp. 1992).
39. Vt. Stat. Ann. tit. 18, sec. 1122 (1982).
40. *Allanson v. Clinton Central School District*, No CV 84-174, slip op. at 5 (N.D.N.Y. 1984).
41. Quoted and cited in Bonnie Miller and Clinton Ray Miller, "Personal Religious Beliefs Are Constitutional Protection Against Compulsory Immunizations," *Health Freedom News*, July-August 1989, p. 35.
42. Ibid.
43. *State Immunization Requirements 1991-1992* (Atlanta: Public Health Service, Centers for Disease Control, 1992), p. 20.

Chapter 15
The Protective Factors In Breast Milk

1. Arnold Goldman and C. Wayne Smith, "Host Resistance Factors In Human Milk," *Journal of Pediatrics* 82, no. 6 (1973): 1083.

2. P. Stanway and A. Stanway, "Breast Milk: The Perfect Food," in *Breast is Best* (Western Publishing Company, 1984), p. 41.

3. Ibid., p. 42.

4. S.S. Ogra and P.L. Ogra, "Immunologic Aspects Of Human Colostrum and Milk," *Journal of Pediatrics* 92, no. 4 (1978): 548.

5. Ibid., p. 546.

6. Ibid., p. 549.

7. Goldman and Wayne, p. 1085.

8. Ibid.

9. Anthony Hayward, "The Immunology of Breast Milk," in *Lactation, Physiology, Nutrition and Breast Feeding*, Margaret Neville and Marianne Neifert, eds., (New York: Plenum Press, 1983), p. 261.

10. Ibid.

11. P. Gyorgy, "A Hitherto Unrecognized Biochemical Difference Between Human Milk and Cow's Milk," *Pediatrics* 11 (1953): 98.

12. Goldman and Wayne, pp. 1082-83.

13. Ibid., p. 1085.

14. Ibid.

15. Ibid.

16. Ibid., p. 1084.

17. Ibid.

18. Ibid.

19. Hayward, p. 257.

20. J.K. Welch and J.T. May, "Anti-Infective Properties Of Breast Milk," *Journal of Pediatrics* 94, no. 1 (1979): 1-9.

21. Albert Sabin and Howard Fieldsteel, "Antipoliomyelitic Activity of Human and Bovine Colostrum and Milk," *Journal of Pediatrics* 29 (1962): 105.

22. Ibid., p. 106.

23. Ibid.

24. Ibid.

25. Ibid., p. 115.

26. Ibid.

180

The author wishes to thank the following for permission to quote or paraphrase material from the sources listed:

Clinical Toxicology of Commercial Products by Robert Gosselin, Roger Smith, and Harold Hodge. Copyright 1984 Williams and Wilkins. Reprinted by permission of the author and publisher; *The Hazards of Immunization* by Sir Graham Wilson. Copyright 1967 University of London. Reprinted by permission of Athlone Press; *American Journal of Public Health*, vol.30, 1940, pp.135-136. Copyright American Public Health Association. Reprinted with permission; *Animal Liberation* by Peter Singer. Copyright 1975 Peter Singer. Reprinted with permission from the *New York Review of Books* and the author; *Immunology: The Science of Self-Non Self Discrimination* by Jan Klein. Copyright 1982 John Wiley and Sons. Used with permission; *The Encyclopedia of Medical Technology* by V.Jegede et al. Copyright 1983 John Wiley and Sons. Reprinted with permission; "Toxic Responses of the Skin," by E.Emmet in *Cassarett and Doull's Toxicology: The Basic Science of Poisons*, 3rd.ed. Copyright 1986 Macmillan Publishing Co. Used with permission; *DPT: A Shot in the Dark* by Harris Coulter and Barbara Loe Fisher. Reprinted with permission of Harris Coulter and Avery Publishing Group, Garden City Park, N.Y.; *Pediatrics*, vol.63 and vol.68 Copyright 1979,1981 *Pediatrics*. Reproduced with permission; *The Case Against Immunizations* by Richard Moskowitz. Copyright 1983 American Institute of Homeopathy. Reprinted by permission of the author and publisher; *Clinical Toxicology*, vol.4, no.2 by M.Mason, C.Cate, and J.Baker. Copyright 1971 Marcel Dekker, Inc. Reprinted courtesy of Marcel Dekker, Inc.; *British Medical Journal*, vol. 2, August 18, 1945, pp.207-08. Used with permission; *American Journal of Hygiene*, vol.13, 1931, pp.296-309 by H.Powell and W.Jamieson; vol.55, 1952, pp.291-300 by J.Younger, E.Ward, and J.Salk; vol.73, 1961, pp.148-163 by J.Bell et al. Reprinted by permission of the *American Journal of Epidemiology*, The John Hopkins University School of Hygiene and Public Health; *The Practical Encyclopedia of Natural Health* by Mark Bricklin. Copyright 1983 by Rodale Press. Permission granted by Rodale Press, Emmaus, PA.; *Essential Immunology*, 2nd ed. by Ivan Roitt. Copyright 1971,1974 Blackwell Scientific Publications. Used with permission; *Journal of the American Medical Association*, vol.251, no.3, 1984, pp.3109-13 by A.Hinman and J.Koplan. Used with permission; JAMA vol.36, no.1, pp.40-41, Copyright 1948 American Medical Association. Used with permission; *Journal of Laboratory and Clinical Medicine*, vol.47, no.1, 1956, pp.8-19 and *Journal of Pediatrics*, vol.29, 1962, pp.105-115; vol.82, no.6, 1973, pp.1082-90. Used by permission of C.V. Mosby Co.

INDEX

A

W

Y

For further reading about the DPT vaccine, the author highly recommends *DPT: A Shot in the Dark* by Harris L. Coulter and Barbara Loe Fisher. This emotionally charged work outlines the history, the adverse reactions, and the political maneuverings behind the most dangerous of the childhood vaccines, DPT. It also contains personal testimonies from parents whose children were injured or killed by the vaccine.

HARRIS L. COULTER, Ph.D., is a respected medical investigator who has written extensively on homeopathy, the history of medicine, and vaccination.

BARBARA LOE FISHER is one of the founding members of Dissatisfied Parents Together, a non-profit educational organization in Vienna, Virginia, which operates the National Vaccine Information Center.

To order *DPT: A Shot in the Dark,* send **$11.50** (check or money order) to:

> Center for Empirical Medicine
> 4221 45th Street, NW
> Washington, D.C. 20016
>
> (202) 364-0898

The **National Vaccine Information Center** is a non-profit, educational organization dedicated to preventing vaccine injuries and deaths through public education. The organization was founded in 1982 by parents whose children died or were injured following vaccination. To learn more about the services they provide, write or call NVIC at:

> National Vaccine Information Center
> 512 W. Maple Avenue #206
> Vienna, Virginia 22180
>
> 1-800-909-7468

Yes, I'd like to order additional copies of **What Every Parent Should Know about Childhood Immunization** by Jamie Murphy. Please send book(s) to:

Name: _____

Address: _____

City: _____

State: _____ Zip: _____

Price: $13.95 per book

Shipping
Parcel Post: $1.75 for the first book, $.75 for each additional book (surface shipping may take three to four weeks).

Air Mail (Priority): $3.50 for the first book, $.75 for each additional book.

Book Trade Orders: please call (508) 385-2055.

Sales Tax: Please add 5% sales tax for books shipped to Massachusetts addresses.

Payment: Make check payable to **Earth Healing Products**, P.O. Box 11-A, Dennis, MA 02638.

Returns/Guarantee: If you are not satisfied with this book, you may return it for a full refund—provided that the book is in good resaleable condition.

ABOUT THE AUTHOR

JAMIE MURPHY is a writer with a long-standing interest in vaccination. He studied natural health at the Ann Wigmore Foundation in Boston and medical herbalism at Gaia Herbal Research Institute in Harvard, Massachusetts. Mr. Murphy lives and works in Massachusetts.